HEALTH
IS
WEALTH

The Art of Healthy Living

By

Gandy Madzalo

ISBN-13: 978-1515369103

ISBN-10: 1515369102

This book is dedicated to all who are willing to learn and to walk along the path of health and wellness which is our valued treasure.

CONTENTS

ACKNOWLEDGMENTS

I'd like to say thank you to my wife Margaret Madzalo and our two daughters Dalitso and Mphatso who share their thinking with me daily, Thomas Schofield, Martha Castañeda, Anne Hillman, Innocent Chitosi and Smith Kalima for their support.

PART I
HEALTH IS WEALTH

1. Introduction

Health is Wealth, without it, the richest man is poor. Driven by passion, my interest in Health and Wellness started 16 years ago. I had chronic eczema – skin diseases. A friend gave me a book on nutrition and I changed my diet – and my eczema disappeared. I then helped a friend who was on TB treatment, who managed to bounce back to health after following a healthy lifestyle and he encouraged me to study Nutritional Medicine as a career. I joined a Nutritional Medicine College in East London, South Africa, in 2002. After working for a number of Wellness Centers and Health Corporations in South Africa till 2008, I decided to be a freelance Wellness educator in my beloved country of Malawi and neighboring countries.

As a Naturopathic Nutritional Therapist, I believe a true physician is an educator, he recognizes his responsibility not only to the sick who are under his care, but also to the community in which he lives. A true healthcare practitioner must inspire, motivate and empower people to live healthier lifestyles and enjoy a measure of good health. When he has done his job, he waits patiently on God to complete the good work in making the man whole.

It does not matter whether you are a carpenter, a business executive, a farmer, a politician or a member of the clergy, we all need health and wellness. Good health is a blessing that many people do not appreciate until they lose it. Wellness, or good health, has traditionally been viewed as being free from disease. Thus, if you were not sick, you were considered healthy. This perspective is changing. While we all agree that the absence of illness is one part of being healthy, it does not indicate whether one is in a state of well-being.

Wellness, as in healthy living, is closely linked with your lifestyle. Each person has a responsibility to provide for such health tools as good nutrition, proper weight control, exercise, and controlling of risk factors such as smoking, alcohol and drug abuse. These things all play a role in wellness. I remember the first time I attended the Wellness health expo in Cape Town, South Africa, in 2005. I had my blood pressure, lung capacity, hydration, body fat, fitness level and health age checked. The best part of it was the stress chair massage that was done on me by one of the practitioners. It was a big surprise when I discovered that I was not as healthy as I thought even though I have always been a "healthy nut" for a big part of my life. My water level was less than normal, something that was placing me at a risk of kidney damage. While my body fat was okay, my fitness level was another major concern. I came out of that expo with new resolutions for my health.

From that day onward I joined the people who

wake up early in the morning going for a 30 minutes to 1 hour walk every day. As a healthcare practitioner I know that if you do not use your legs you will finally lose them. This is true especially if you end up becoming a diabetic because of a sedentary lifestyle. You may end up having the legs amputated due to uncontrolled blood sugar. If you happen to have blood pressure issues it is not something better either. Stroke may follow, leaving you incapacitated and failing to use your legs one more time. Walk while you can. Drinking eight glasses of water every day between meals is not just a good habit but it works just as well as medicine. In some cases it is ten times better than a pile of tablets. Drinking enough water every day is now part of my religion, thanks to the Wellness health expo I attended back then. Wellness is not the mere absence of diseases. It is a proactive, preventive approach designed to achieve optimum levels of health.

A wellness-oriented lifestyle encourages you to adopt habits and behaviors that promote better health and an improved quality of life. It also involves the recognition that you have physical, psychological, social and spiritual needs, with each dimension being necessary for optimal levels of functioning. Wellness is a positive approach to living – an approach that emphasizes the whole person. It is the integration of the body, mind, and spirit; and the appreciation that everything you do, think, feel, and believe has an impact on your state of health. Health is treasury; of all temporary blessings that we have in this life nothing can surpass good health. We appreciate everything that we have only when we have a measure of good health. Education and riches are nothing if wellness is missing. Remember wellness is a life-long process of moving towards enhancing your physical, intellectual, emotional, social, spiritual, and environmental well-being. Take time to explore your own level of wellness and see if you got "your dose of wellness" today!

Since lifestyle has been found to be the single most important factor determining your pattern of general health, it is important that you be educated to take charge of your daily life and to set healthy lifestyle goals. Many people think that it is the job of a medical doctor to fix them up when they are sick. The truth of the matter is that as medical professionals we may provide good treatment for various diseases but we cannot give you good health. ***Seeing a medical practitioner when you are sick*** is increasingly important for early detection of serious illnesses and conditions. However there needs to be a greater emphasis on the ***prevention of lifestyle diseases.*** Health is a choice. The choices you make may have a dominant influence on your health and wellness. The secret is not in medical care, but consistent self-care. While traditionally medicine concentrates on alleviating or curing diseases, the wellness approach encourages you to take personal responsibility for your well-being.

2. Start from the Beginning

Many people think that the older you grow the more conscious you should become of what you eat or the way you live. They believe that as a child or as long as you are young, there is no need to deny yourself the so-called pleasures that come as a result of indulgence in eating and lifestyle habits. But we can always learn from the farmers. Every farmer knows that if they do not look after their plants from the nursery bed, they will mess up the quality of those plants for good. Even if they apply fertilizer at a later stage, the quality will still be compromised. The same principle applies to us human beings. If we do not look after our kids starting from the womb, after birth and during the growing years, their health will be compromised throughout life. We all know of kids who have learning difficulties just because their mothers or fathers were consuming a lot of alcohol either before conception (in case of fathers) or when expecting them.

Conceiving a baby – the sowing time

Only good seeds can produce good crops. Good nutrition and healthy lifestyle practices are crucial even before conception. How you look after your health as a mother and even a father before you decide to have a child matters a lot to the health of the offspring. If a father is an alcoholic or smokes cigarettes, that affects the fruit of the womb. The same applies if the mother enjoys her alcoholic drinks or smokes, especially during pregnancy. Poor nutrition can affect mental development of the child in the womb as well as the general growth of the child. Intelligent kids are fed well, starting in the womb. The quality of foods the mother eats is exactly what the baby will get. No miracles will happen in the mother's stomach if she eats junk food during pregnancy.

It is sad sometimes to see an expectant mother having a feast of fried chips and fizzy drinks as a meal at lunch time. While the fizzy drink may cool your throat, it is not a cool diet for the baby growing in your body. The baby needs nourishment that comes from dark green vegetables, even better if you add nuts and seeds to them. It is a time when you should eat more fruits and whole grains like nobody's business. The whole grains will give you more of the B vitamins needed for all functions of developing a healthy baby. They are also packed with complex carbohydrates which will provide sustainable energy for you and the baby. Corn flour, brown rice, oats, baked potato and whole wheat products are the best examples of complex carbohydrates. A few almonds three times per week will provide the unborn baby with lecithin (brain nutrients). Avocado, pears and nuts will provide your baby with the essential fats required for hormones, immune system and brain development and do not forget the beans family (legumes) which is rich in minerals.

On the contrary, a diet high in cholesterol and refined foods may predispose the unborn baby to risk factors of chronic conditions like diabetes, high blood pressure and cancer. The more natural the diet the healthier the baby will be, and if you add to that better lifestyle practices like avoiding smoking, alcohol, fizzy drinks, refined food and caffeinated drinks or foods before and during pregnancy, the chances for you to have a super kid will be very high. What you sow today is exactly what you will reap. That is the 'law of harvest'.

Diet of a new-born baby – the weeding time

Experiencing birth is one of the great wonders in life; bringing life to Earth is more amazing than the so-called seven wonders of the earth. It confirms what the Scriptures state "we are fearfully and wonderfully made" – Psalms 139:14. Every married woman cannot wait to have this experience at least once in life. Now that you have a baby, please remember that nature has already provided a diet for the child for the first six months – and that is breast milk. Ever wonder that wild or domestic animals do not give milk of another animal to their offspring? Human beings are the only strange species on planet Earth that experiment with the life of their babies by giving them milk of other species. Exclusive breast feeding means the mother should feed the child breast milk only with no other foods or fluids, not even water during the first six months of a child's life, unless advised otherwise by a recognised health professional. Breast milk from the mother is rich in growth hormones, immune system nutrients and prevents the child from contracting a number of illnesses. Studies have also shown that by breast feeding your baby, you may lower the child's risk of developing diabetes type 1, lung diseases and many chronic conditions. Of course the best breast milk will come as a result of the healthy diet of the mother. You need to weed out all the junk we see in town for the sake of your child's health. That is the way to start healthy living.

3. Child Obesity

A Pressure Cooker

The problem of child obesity is now part of the health crisis in our urban areas. In my clinical practice, I have consulted children as young as 11 years weighing over 120 kilogrammes. Overweight to some parents is considered as a symbol of a good life. Some mothers think if their two-year-old baby is weighing 25 kilogrammes, it means he or she qualifies as baby of the week. Indeed, very few parents in our time understand that allowing children to become overweight is like putting the health of the child in a pressure cooker.

These overweight children can easily suffer from non-communicable diseases of lifestyle like developing illnesses such as high blood pressure (hypertension), pre-diabetes, diabetes, heart disease, high cholesterol, sleeping problems, breathing problems, bone conditions such as weakening of the hips, gastro-intestinal diseases, and even the early onset of puberty. There are also psychological complications to consider, with many obese children suffering from poor self-esteem and depression. In fact, most obese children develop high blood pressure at a very young age.

The cost of inactivity

But who is to blame for these overweight kids we have in our homes? And, the problem is even becoming worse in developing countries. Many Africans, and those in other parts of the developing world, will recall the good old days when we grew up. Life was full of activities. We had to do manual work at home before going to school only to be welcomed by more manual work at school before starting classes. We knew all the names of the garden tools as early as in standard 1. All games were played outdoors, playing soccer made from a pile of plastic bags, skipping ropes and pushing old bicycle rims were among some of the exciting daily games that we played. You may remember coming home late in the day full of dust and you had to bathe in cold water. Now, what have we done to our kids today? We are encouraging a sedentary lifestyle at a very young age. Unlike our youth, the children of today spend their time watching cartoons, sitting with PlayStations, watching games instead of playing them the way we did. If parents are blessed with more cash they send the kids to the so-called better schools where no manual work is taught to their children. Furthermore, as is the case in many other parts of the world, children who play computer games, or sit in front of the TV all day long, do not get any exercise and thus their bodies do not burn as much energy as they should. Then we wonder why our children are getting so big and often getting ill raising the cost on family medical bills.

The junk food syndrome

In addition to the lack of exercise, we are feeding our children with highly processed foods either out of convenience or simply because as parents we do not know any better. For those of us who grew up in developing countries, our diet was simple. Cornflour porridge with groundnut flour for breakfast, sweet potatoes or cassava on lucky days and we had to snack on all fruits in season whether it was bananas, baobab fruit, mango, tamarind, guavas, granadillas, berries, not to mention sugar cane, which was like our natural toothbrush. We were proud to carry roasted maize filled in a used cooking oil bottle to school. I do not need to remind you that we were very strong kids back then. These days a 15-year-old kid cannot do the manual work that we did at a tender age of 10.

Today, we are feeding our kids ice cream, cheese, excessive animal fats, all the high salts, highly processed junk foods, cakes and fizzy drinks available in town. Modern parents think they are doing their children a favour by exposing them to this deadly lifestyle. Sometimes we are tempted to think that we grew up during the time of trouble, and now that we have enough disposable income we need to offer our children a good life. Unfortunately, it is the good life that is killing our kids.

From this day onward

It is high time we went back to the basics of healthy living. Of course, in this age we do not expect our children to carry roasted maize in used bottles of cooking oil to school, but we can always give them something better. Some boiled or baked potatoes with onion and tomato instead of fried chips can make a good school lunch box. You may add a banana and an apple with some nuts. Bake some home made whole wheat rolls or banana muffins to replace the junk cakes and biscuits. Provide whole fruit juices instead of fizzy drinks. Do not buy toys that will encourage a sedentary lifestyle, rather buy toys such as bicycles, or even better, some gardening tools for your child to use at home. Always teach by example. If you ask a child of today to go and work in the garden it will prove to be difficult, but as a parent if you go together with your son or daughter to work in the garden it will be much easier. Make small changes at a time and it will soon become a lifestyle.

4. Raising Super Kids

Our parents used to be proud of their children's ability in learning things and skills early in life. The children who demonstrated a better level of intelligence as compared to their age-mates were considered as super kids. But today things have changed. Instead of super kids, we are proud of super-size kids. Raising healthy kids is a choice, not a chance. It is sad to see modern parents leaving the health of their little ones to the mercies of their home maids, who in most cases understand very little about good health.

We should always remember that the first five years are precious in your child's life. Poor growth at this stage of life can have life-long consequences. This is the time the brain of your child develops to its full capacity. You may have observed that kids under five years can learn a number of languages and speak all of them fluently with ease. As you get older learning a new language is never the easiest adventure. It is also the time they develop resistance to many illnesses if their immune system is well fed.

Feeding the young mind

The growing brain needs a good supply of energy from complex carbohydrates. The best sources are wholegrain cereals like oat porridge, millet or sorghum with soya porridge or some whole wheat bran. Adding whole fruits to their breakfast like a banana, apple, orange or fruit in season will make the day for them. Remember they also need healthy fats found in avocados, olives, seeds and nuts. If you are a mother who enjoys baking, you may grind some sunflower and flax seeds as well as adding them to your home made whole wheat fruity muffins. Your child can carry this yummy muffin with a fruit or a 100 percent fruit juice to school. Pumpkin seeds are high in zinc, a well-known brain nutrient. Some people even say that zinc is for thinking. Giving your kids pumpkin seeds to chew is a non-starter. The best way is to grind them and add to whole fruit smoothies blended with soya milk. It is delicious and more nutritious than fruit juices.

Add more fibre to the lunch

Adding food high in fibre in your children's lunch will lower the risk of obesity. Fibre is the functional carbohydrate which absorbs excess glucose and cholesterol from your digestive system. It is naturally found in unprocessed plant based foods. The best sources are legumes like beans, lentils, pigeon peas, cow peas, mung beans, etc. Among the grains, brown rice and whole wheat are the leaders. Fruits and vegetables contain a little fibre as well but cannot beat that of legumes and grains. The habit of eating fibre early in life also lowers the risk of developing diabetes and blood pressure throughout life. Foods high in fibre are also rich in vitamins, minerals, proteins and other essential trace elements usually found in whole foods. Because fibre fills the tummy, it helps your child not to join the group of grazing kids – children who eat all day long.

Cut down on junk food

It is common knowledge that health food cannot compete with junk food when it comes to tempting the taste buds. A wise parent will avoid supplying their kids with junk food. The best way is simply not to buy them. The more kids are exposed to junk food the less they will enjoy the healthier options. The evils of junk food are not just poor nutrition. The chemicals added to these processed foods are now known to have the potential to weaken children's immune system. Have you ever wondered why, when you were growing, you were eating all the fruits in season from tamarind to baobab and you mainly lived on a natural diet – even though you were exposed to a lot of infections you hardly got sick? But look at our kids today, living the good life we still have to take them to expensive hospitals every Monday. That tells us something has gone amiss with the immune system.

Water, water everywhere

Remember the body is made of water; we have water everywhere. Let a child learn early in life the habit of drinking lots of pure water. It is sad to see more kids today who will refuse to drink anything if it does not have colour. But remember kids learn by observing. What you do as a parent they believe that is what they must do. If they see you drinking lots of water, they will cry for it too.

5. TV & Children's Health

Television can be a source of education and clean entertainment or it can negatively impact your child's mental and spiritual health. As a responsible parent it is important to be vigilant about what your child watches and the amount of time they spend watching television. Good programs are available, such as the History Channel or National Geographic, selected good spiritual channels to enlighten the child's mind on the topics of science, history, nature, religion, art and human interest.

I learnt about the danger of television to children's health some years ago when I was staying with friends, where I noticed that their children sat in front of the screen for hours at a time. The parents usually had great difficulty in persuading them to come to the table to eat or go to bed and they lost interest in family worship. The negative effects of this abnormal behaviour were disturbing, difficult to combat and overcome. The children were in an overwrought state, with a poor appetite, their school achievements had dropped, they were absent minded, lacked concentration and were much more subject to infectious diseases. Indeed, even at such a young age their health had already been undermined.

Advantages of television

Television is one of the modern day inventions that most of us cannot imagine being without. This is no exaggeration, no sooner had it cast its spell when people rush out to buy one, whether it is necessary or not. Of course, TV in moderation can be a good thing. Pre-school children can get help learning the alphabet on a home television, primary pupils can learn about wildlife on nature shows, and parents can keep up with current events. There are also a number of spiritual channels to enrich our families with spiritual manna. No doubt about it – TV can be an excellent educator and entertainer. But despite its advantages, too much television watching can be detrimental especially to children's wellness: The horror graphics and violent scenes in most so-called kids' TV programs stimulate and increase stress-hormone production in the brain. Take note of any signs of anxiety, mood swings, aggression or violence in children. It is of vital importance that you protect the impressionable mind of your child.

Modern day parenting

During the years when I was growing up, parenting was a serious business. Parents who owned video sets back then were highly selective in the choice of intellectual nourishment for their children's minds. In those days a video set used to be in a locked cabinet and the keys were on the bunch of parents' office keys, meaning that children could not watch the video unless their parents were at home. Parents only were making choices about what type of movies could be watched and for how long. But today we see busy fathers and civilized mothers in high heels, are using a TV as an assistant parent to their kids, because they do not have time for the little ones. To make it worse, some parents think that violent and abusive movies, or computer games, are harmless. Remember children learn behaviour by observing. What they absorb through watching is recorded in their subconscious brain and it becomes part of them. It's like programming a computer to do certain tasks.

The effects of too much screen time

The American Academy of Pediatrics recommends limiting a child's use of TV, movies, video and computer games to no more than one or two hours a day. Children who consistently spend more than four hours per day watching TV are more likely to be overweight. TV characters often depict risky behaviours, such as smoking and drinking. Primary school students who have TVs in their bedrooms tend to perform worse in school than those who do not. Too much exposure to violence on TV and in movies, music videos, computer and video games can desensitize children to violence. As a result, children may learn to accept violent behaviour as a normal part of life and a way to solve problems. That is why it is so important for parents to monitor the content of TV programmes and set viewing limits to ensure that kids do not spend too much time in front of the TV. Obesity, diabetes, heart disease and hypertension in children are linked to too much TV viewing. This behaviour encourages a sedentary lifestyle and too much intake of junk food like ice cream, fizzy drinks, cakes, etc. If kids are going to bed late their immune system is suppressed, hence they can easily suffer from infections.

How to limit screen time

It is possible to take simple steps to reduce the amount of time your child spends watching TV, movies and videos or playing video or computer games: Keep TVs and computers out of the bedroom. Children who have TVs in their bedrooms watch more TV and videos than children who do not. Monitor your child's screen time and the websites he or she is visiting by keeping computers in a common area in your house. Do not eat in front of the TV because it increases children's screen time. The habit also encourages mindless grazing, which can lead to overeating and weight gain. Suggest other activities rather than relying on screen time for entertainment; consider alternative activities, such as reading, playing a musical instrument, swimming or trying some outdoor games. As a parent, set a good example. Be a good role model by limiting your own screen time.

6. How to Have a Healthy Pregnancy

God gave women a very special role – the ability to carry in their bodies the future generations of this world. This is not an easy task. Pregnant women need special care from their partners, families and communities. A woman's body changes a lot during pregnancy. Another person is living inside her. She will need more food, more rest, and more love than before. Anything that could hurt her body may also hurt the baby.

A pregnant woman needs to eat well to have the strength to work, fight illness, and stay healthy. Eating well protects the mother's teeth and bones and makes the baby grow strong in her womb. She will be stronger at the time she gives birth and will have less bleeding. Eating well during pregnancy helps the mother to fight infections and to recover quickly after the baby is born. Good food will also help her to have plenty of milk for breast-feeding. Whole grains, legumes, nuts, seeds fruits and vegetables form the ideal diet during pregnancy. These main foods should not be refined or polished because then much of the goodness is destroyed. For example, whole wheat bread is better than white bread and brown rice is better than white rice. Other food supplements like dark molasses are a good source of vitamins and minerals.

Apart from eating well, there are many other important things we can do. Keeping clean is very important in staying healthy during pregnancy. Bathe and wash regularly, and brush your teeth every day. Keeping clean will help prevent infections. Be active. In rural places women get all the exercise they need by carrying water, working in the fields, milling grain, and walking up and down hills. Women who work in the office need to have time for exercise. Walking is the best.

Rest is just us good during pregnancy. Rest helps pregnant women to stay strong and fight against illnesses. It also helps prevent miscarriages, high blood pressure, sick babies and other problems. Eight hours of good sleep each night is best.

It is good for a pregnant woman to sit and relax a little every few hours, put her feet up, or even take a short nap. The family needs to know and understand that it is important for her to rest, even during the day.

Do not drink alcohol. Alcohol can cause a baby to be deformed, and have a head and brain that is too small. Because of this, the baby might be slow mentally. A woman who drinks alcohol may also not eat as well as she should. This can lead to more health problems for her and the unborn baby.

Avoid smoking or sitting closer to someone who is smoking. Passive smoking can equally do harm. Smoking is especially harmful to pregnant mothers. It causes her blood vessels to get smaller. As a result, less food and air are carried to the baby in her womb. The baby starves and cannot grow properly. It might even become ill and die in the womb.

Coffee, tea, and cola drinks contain caffeine. Caffeine can damage the nerves of the baby. As the child grows, it may become too active and not be able to concentrate well. It may have difficulty learning things at school. It would be best for all women to avoid these harmful things, because most women do not find out that they are pregnant until the second month of pregnancy. By that time, damage may have already been done to their baby.

7. Preventing Pimples During Adolescence

Known as acne in healthcare, it is a condition consisting of pimples usually prominent on the cheeks and chin, or other parts of the face as well as the chest, shoulders, and back. Acne usually runs its course in 10-15 years, and often leaves the face smooth, but sometimes pockmarked. It is not unusual to see people who are more than 21 years old to have pimples as well.

Acne is usually common during the adolescent years when the oil glands of the skin go through an extended period of active development like the rest of the glands of the body. This may cause them to develop sensitivity and an overgrowth in susceptible persons. In this case the oil glands become clogged, swollen and inflamed. They are prone to infection. The cystic form of acne can be disfiguring and include chronic, widespread, large and painful lumps. Pimples, red spots, blackheads and whiteheads, swollen areas on the face, chest, shoulders and back usually occur just at the time in life when social relationships are the most important, and looking good is highly desirable.

One way to help an adolescent avoid the development of acne is by promoting slow and steady growth in children, rather than the explosive growth often seen at puberty in our cities today. This is done by a lifetime of a healthful diet and lifestyle. Slow down the growth of children if they are the tallest, fattest, or biggest compared with the average on growth charts by putting them on a moderate whole food diet. Cut down animal products which are known to have a concentrate of growth hormones due to modern farming practices.

Diet

A whole food plant-based diet will be found to be most helpful, eating fruits and vegetables, whole grains like brown rice and whole wheat bread freely. Eat nuts sparingly but enjoy liberally all foods richly coloured green or yellow. Cut down on sugar, fizzy drinks and highly refined foods. Do not mix too many foods in one meal. Besides being stimulating to the appetite, it causes chemical warfare inside you. Keep dishes and menus simple. Avoid becoming overweight or overeating. Being overweight stimulates the production of hormones that contribute to acne. Overeating encourages "leaky gut" (damaged small intestines) which has become a suspect in a wide variety of disorders, including skin diseases in recent years. Avoid constipation by proper measures. Fast one day weekly.

PART II
EAT WELL

8. *The Cost of Eating Unhealthily*

Many people believe that it is expensive to eat healthy. Well, maybe it depends on where you are. However in most places around the world the opposite is true. Many countries are rich in a wide variety of indigenous nutritious foods. Just take a walk to any local food market today. You will find a wide variety of foods in season. In fact in our cities you will find almost in every street some shop selling some locally grown or imported foods.

Our rich food basket

During the good old days in many countries people enjoyed eating a wide variety of foods. People were eating almost anything that could be eaten. From the bush fruits to indigenous grains, nothing was spared. You think of baobab fruit, millet, sorghum, brown rice, strawberries, kiwi fruit, grapefruit and many bush vegetables, fruits which today we can hardly find due to deforestation. But not everything is lost. We still have lots of nutritious foods in our food markets. Pumpkins are still greeting our tables, talk of the yummy avocados. Organic sweet potatoes, which are sweet not just in name, but they taste really sweet.

Save money, stay healthy

It's not just good for our bodies to eat healthy, it is cheaper as well. One day I was talking with one of my diabetic patients who successfully managed to stabilize his blood sugar through a healthy diet and lifestyle we prescribed to him. When I asked him, what was the first thing he noticed when he started the healthy eating plan his reply was, "My food budget went down by half." We can all agree with him. Every time I visit our local food markets, I find healthy foods much cheaper compared to others. Compare the cost of beans with high fat meats which today we know these fatty foods to be the mothers of our chronic diseases. Think of spinach, broccoli, cauliflower, beetroot, pumpkin leaves, sweet potato leaves, and cassava leaves – you don't need to be a dietician to know that these foods are nutritious. Yet they are much cheaper compared to their cousins like Chinese rape etc. The time when most people eat the healthiest is when they are poor. Go to the African villages today, people are eating everything from sorghum, to organic bush vegetables garnished with groundnuts flour. All root vegetables are eaten without mercy and the fruits in season are the desserts, what a feast of good nutrition.

The cost of an unhealthy diet

Eating unhealthy will not just empty your wallet but it will also compromise your total well-being. I mean, it is costly to have a breakfast of two sausages, two eggs, some cheese, dip fried chips, a cup of strong coffee plus bread with jam. Compare that with the cost of Cooked Oats cereal with soya milk, or some mashed sweet potato with groundnut flour and some fruits kind of a breakfast – a big money saver. But that's not all; a diet high in fat is a risk factor for heart diseases, diabetes, stroke, kidney failure, some cancers, etc. You pay heavily for these foods and you spend all your savings trying to manage the curses that come with them. The so-called good refined junk foods are killing us.

9. Planning Healthy Meals

Many people are interested to start eating healthy. But just to be interested is not enough; we need to start doing something about it. A healthy diet is one that helps maintain or improve general health. A balanced nutrition adequate in fluids, body building nutrients, healthy fats, vitamins, minerals, and the major source of energy – calories – is what we need.

Planning healthy meals can be difficult, especially if your family is stuck in a rut of eating unhealthy meals. However, with some basic knowledge of nutrition, you can have your family eating healthy without them even realising it. The key to creating healthy meals is to plan. Plan your week's meals ahead of time so that you have all of the necessary ingredients. Do not let a lack of ingredients stop you. Be creative in the kitchen and try to invent some new ways of preparing food with what you have.

While shopping, get only the foods that are on your list and stay away from the junk food aisles to limit temptation. This will also allow you to keep your food costs to a minimum. Make sure you do much of your shopping from local food markets where you can easily get a wider variety of fruits and vegetables fresh from the garden.

Make it quick

Huge time savers are pre-cooked foods. This does not suggest that you should buy pre-cooked foods. But during weekends or off days when you are at home, you can cook a lot of legumes and store them in the fridge. If you enjoy baking you can get your healthy bread, carrot muffins, etc. done. The same principle can be done with a variety of foods like rice, etc. This will save time during meal preparation. All you will need is to take the frozen beans, warm them and mix them with a healthy, freshly made sauce or gravy. You can prepare some foods once a week and split them for the rest of the week. A slow cooker, if available, will allow foods to cook all day while you are at work. When you get home, a delicious and healthy meal will be waiting for you.

Get the family involved

Do not just prescribe a healthy diet to your family. First share your desire and passion for healthy eating and how it will work for the good of the whole family. Eating healthily is a family affair. It is important to get everyone in the family involved so that each member's preferences are considered. You do not want anyone to feel as though they are being deprived of their choices. If possible, get the whole family involved in the cooking. This allows children to learn their way around the kitchen and recognize what ingredients are healthy.

Stock up on healthy foods

It is impossible to prepare healthy meals if you do not stock up on healthy ingredients in your kitchen. Even better, you may empty your kitchen of all unhealthy food stuffs to avoid the temptation of using them. Eating healthy should not be expensive. In fact it is a money saving exercise. When you are buying the grains or grain products, try your best to get only the wholegrain products. These may include items like whole wheat flour, whole maize flour, whole wheat pasta, brown rice, etc. Other food stuffs like tomatoes, onions and vegetables can be sourced cheaply in some specific local markets, rather than the usual produce markets. It is wise to locate where specific foods are cheaper and if means allow, buy in bulk those food items that you can manage to preserve. Get healthy spices, usually these are food-based spices like garlic, ginger, coriander, green pepper, paprika, lemon juice, etc. Try to avoid chemical-based spices.

Make it fun

Do not give your family the same food item everyday just because it is healthy. Even though we know that a bran muffin can lower your cholesterol, it does not mean it should be your daily bread. Your kids will soon have enough of it and they may boycott your healthy menu. Add variety to your menu, make it fun. You can have some fruits today and make a fruit salad tomorrow. Done wisely your family will wonder why you never did this before. Eat well and live well.

10. The Wholegrain Diet

The story of whole grains may not hit the headlines but it is one of the key points we need to understand about nutrition and health. Whole grains are packed with nutrients that are the key to long lasting weight loss and super health, helping to counter heart disease, diabetes and other conditions. Forget fad diets; eating whole grains is the scientifically proven way to improve health and vitality. In my clinical practice, I have found that almost everybody who suffers from dietary-related disease is actually feasting on refined grains. Even those who claim to be eating healthy still need to be converted to adopt a whole grain diet.

The way we eat fresh maize, that's how God intended that we should eat the grains. Remember the story of creation when God finished creating something he signed his signature under it by saying, "it is good", meaning that it is good for you and me. We are supposed to eat everything from the grain. Every time you eat fresh maize, you eat it together with the fibre and the yellow germ which is rich in vitamin E. The whole grain is also rich in vitamins and minerals. I feel sad to see millions of people worldwide who are, either by choice or ignorance, denying themselves all the goodies from the whole grains like brown rice, whole wheat, whole millet, whole sorghum, etc. To make it worse, in some cultures we have stigmatized the whole grain flour as a symbol of poverty. If a pastor comes to my home and he finds me attacking my brown rice or whole maize flour pulp with legumes and some local vegetables, he will be tempted to start praying for financial breakthroughs for me. He may hardly believe that I am eating that way by choice, just for the health of it. In fact we always give the best to animals. Animal food is better looked after than human food. When we refine the grain, the germ and the fibre are given to the pigs and chickens, no wonder our animals are very healthy and we are very sick.

Sometimes in some African cultures, if the food makers are cruel enough, they will soak the refined grain (mphale) in water for three or four days to come up with pure, or what they may call, supper white maize flour. The soaking water (ntombera) that we throw away or give to animals is rich in B vitamins and some trace minerals. These vitamins are crucial for the normal functioning of the brain, the immune system, the digestion system, among other functions. A brain with less B vitamins will function like a Pentium one computer with a slow processor. You struggle to remember a thing, that's the time you start calling everybody my elder – simply because you can't remember their names and you are ashamed to ask them over and over again.

The same principal applies to all the grains, whether it's wheat, sorghum, millet or rice. The more whole the grain, the better it is for our health. The more we demand these healthy whole grains the more we will find these foods in our local markets. The food sellers work on the principal of demand, they sell what we consume. Today we find a lot of brown rice in most super markets in town, something which was considered a sin 10 years ago. If this trend continues, we are heading in the right direction.

Furthermore, the whole grains are rich in functional carbohydrates known as fibre. We don't absorb fibre into our systems the way we do other nutrients. But as fibre passes your digestive system it works like a broom sweeping all the waste in your small and large intestines by preventing chronic conditions like piles and colon cancers. Whole grains absorb the excess glucose in your meal, lowering your risk of diabetes. Even your heart smiles when you have more whole grains in your meal because it lowers excess cholesterol – the fat that kills.

All the patients I have assisted in eliminating gall stones naturally without the use of surgery were all white flour product eaters. The whole grain absorbs bile from your small intestines and that activity prevents the formation of gall bladder stones. The trace minerals like zinc and selenium found in whole grains are crucial for the male reproductive system. They are a secret for the fountain of youth. Germ in the whole grain lowers the risk of most cancers like breast cancer, liver cancer and prostate cancer. For all these reasons, that's why I eat whole grains at my home and you can do it too.

11. *Natural Diet and Health*

Many of us have heard a lot of a natural diet. But what is a natural diet? A good natural diet consists partly of cooked and partly of raw foods. In today's living environment, it is certainly difficult for the home makers to feed their families along scientific lines. Even an expert in the field of diet and nutrition would find it difficult to prepare a diet which takes into consideration calories, minerals, proteins, fats, vitamins and trace elements in their required amounts and qualities. While some guidelines of healthy eating can be helpful, our personal nutritional needs may differ from one person to another due to the status of each individual's health. Sometimes due to our past dietary habits we lose the ability to digest raw foods. Such individuals should begin with small quantities of raw juices first and gradually increase them. Then start taking small amounts of finely grated raw vegetables and fruit. Increase the intake of these until you are once more able to eat the foods in their natural state. Cutting off junk food will also help our taste buds to start appreciating the natural flavours of raw foods. If there is no need to change over to an exclusively raw food diet, as with some sickness, nevertheless, it would be beneficial for all of us to incorporate small quantities in our daily meals. Especially those foods that can be eaten raw, we should try to eat them like that. Learn the art of making delicious fruits and vegetable salads seasoned with medicinal herbs.

Vegetables and fruits should not be taken at the same meal, but be taken separately. If you break this rule you are likely to be bothered with digestive problems like flatulence. Experience has proved that most people will do better if they keep these two foods apart and today's nutrition science agrees with this principle. Our taste buds would hardly find a mixture of broccoli or cauliflower and strawberries acceptable. Remember, the health value of vegetables depends upon the soil in which they are grown. Sick soil will produce sick plants. That is why home gardens are always encouraged because it is very important to grow our own fruits and vegetables organically. That art of growing your own vegetables provides an opportunity to do physical activities for better physical and mental health. Much is being taught nowadays about organic farming which includes: biological soil cultivation, compost gardening, biodynamic soil health, among others. Take advantage of the indigenous vegetables as most of them grow without the aid of chemicals.

Eating food closer to its natural state, prepared in a much simpler way instead of depending on refined processed foods, is a major step in healthy eating. Primitive people are more sensible than we are in this respect. They take their food just as it grows and prepare it very simply, thus preserving its nutritive value. How we prepare the food in the kitchen matters. Most healthy foods are destroyed in the kitchen through poor cooking methods. More processed foods are being invented every day either at home or by food manufacturing companies, but do we see a decline in the incidence of diseases generally? Far from it, many people are dying from dietary related diseases which we sometimes call the "eating well syndrome". The thing is that most of us have confused the eating of junk food with civilisation, or a status symbol. Certain diseases are becoming more prevalent than ever, especially those that are connected with diet and poor lifestyle practices. Among the most notable are cancer, diabetes, and high blood pressure. Degenerative changes in the cells of the body, in most people today, occur chiefly among those who live on highly refined and processed foods.

It is only whole food that offers real substance and protection. Everything offered by nature consists of an integral whole and if, through human folly, only a fraction is used, whatever it may be, we are deprived of something that would otherwise provide us with complete nutrition.

Foods, canned or tinned, cannot be recommended under any circumstance, if the fresh equivalent is available. Maybe they are foods to be used in times of emergencies. They are better than starving but they come with their shortfalls as well from the nutrition point of view. These foods are treated with so many chemical additions; most of them are heavily refined and deprived of most of their health-giving elements, that there is no place for them in a natural healthy diet. Home canned foods are probably less harmful and can be tolerated when there is no availability of fresh foods and thus they would be a supplement to the usual fare. By this time it should be self-evident that a practical, healthy diet should consist of whole natural foods in as close to their natural state as possible. Various diseases will disappear without medication of any sort, if we feed our bodies with the best fuel it needs to function optimally.

12. Diets: Quick Fix Traps

Many people today want to lose weight and they want to lose it now. Yes, we are living in the age of instant coffee, instant money transfer, instant transport, etc. But when it comes to weight loss, a gentle and gradual natural way is the best. I have seen a lot of people who jump from one diet to another trying to lose weight now, only to gain it back later. Experience shows that this swing effect gradually depletes important body tissues such as muscle and bone. Eventually it weakens the body so that it becomes more susceptible to disease and less able to shed excess fat. Some quick fixes can even damage some essential organs like liver and kidneys. But, being fat or overweight is obviously not healthy as it's one of the risk factors of chronic diseases. Excess weight impairs health and shortens life. As little as five to ten kilogrammes of extra weight produce measurable changes that can lay the foundation for degenerative diseases and for every five kilogrammes you are overweight, the life span can be shortened by as much as one year.

Diets do not work

You do not need a new diet. You do need a new dietary lifestyle. You may seem to lose some weight after going through that cabbage soup diet. But within days, when you resume to your former eating pattern, you will gain back all the weight. People who are overweight need major revisions in thinking and attitudes. Stop the blame game and change your lifestyle. Weight control diets usually fail because they are short-term fixes for long-term problems. It is time to face reality that obesity can be a serious and life threatening condition. Managing obesity is much more than a dietary problem. Like diabetes, hypertension, alcoholism, or smoking, obesity requires a holistic approach to dietary and lifestyle change.

No magic pills

Have you ever asked yourself a question; how do we gain weight in the first place? It's easy to find the solution if we understand the underlying cause of the problem. The dream of many people is a magic pill that will remove all the fat in the body. In the absence of such a magic pill, we continue to try dozens of diets, spend a fortune on exercise equipment and health club membership, we read so much about what is good for us and what is bad to a point of getting of confused of the whole picture. Trying to learn about weight loss through adverts is a bad school. Advertising these days is so sleek and full of deception that we often do not know what to believe anymore.

Take the long-term approach

It is virtually impossible to lose weight and keep it off if you do not modify your lifestyle. Make eating the right foods a permanent part of your daily life. This is a solution to being overweight. Don't go on a diet but start a new lifestyle and live a happier, healthier life. Ask yourself some great questions: can you make a long-term commitment to the new lifestyle? Are you willing to bypass the seductive offers of diets that claim to melt the kilogrammes away in a few days, instead of focusing on good health? The real risk comes when people eat a lot of fatty foods and load up on sweets and other refined foods and snacks instead of eating more real foods, such as oatmeal, brown rice, potatoes with the skin, legumes, fruits and vegetables. Avoid meats, sausages, eggs and dairy products, fatty sauces, margarines, butter and mayonnaise. Use natural herbs like ginger and garlic with healthy fats like olive oil. Limit sugar, syrups, pies, cakes, biscuits, soft drinks, and sugar-rich desserts, like pudding and ice cream. Avoid alcohol and caffeinated beverages such as coffee, colas and black tea.

A balanced lifestyle

Live a balanced life and avoid extremes. Eating healthy does not mean you need to be a fanatic. Make time for work, play, rest, exercise and hobbies. Always try to reserve seven to eight hours a night for rest and sleep. The earlier you go to bed the more fat you are likely to burn while resting. Lighten your body's metabolic load and increase circulation by drinking plenty of water – at least eight glasses per day between meals. Never forget physical activities like walking, cycling, swimming or working outdoors. You need to jumpstart your day with a whole grain and fruits breakfast. Eating healthy may make your eating habits different from those of your peers. It is okay to be different, especially if you are doing it for your health and wellness.

13. The Healing Fats

Many people today are becoming health conscious. That means they are careful about what they eat, drink, etc. Some have even decided not to eat any fat in order to preserve their health or to maintain their normal body weight. Others even wonder if they should be eating fat at all. What we need is not low fat, no fat or fake fat. We need the right fats in our diet.

Some fats kill and some fats heal; this is the first thing we need to understand about fats. If you want to be healthy know the difference between the bad and the good. Some fats promote cancer, other fats inhibit cancer, and some fats inhibit immune function. Other fats are required for and enhance our immune system. Some fats make us more susceptible to a stroke or a heart attack. Other fats protect us from heart attacks and strokes. Some fats may interfere with mental health, while other fats are crucial for brain development and function. These good fats are also extremely important for the health of women, especially during pregnancies and throughout their life circle.

Fats and cancer

We are living at a time when cases of cancer are now becoming a pandemic, among other risk factors like smoking, alcohol, hormones, obesity, and others. For example, re-using of refined cooking oils, either at home or from vendors like restaurants and the popular street take-away, is a great risk factor for cancer. Refined cooking oils are not supposed to be used twice. In fact deep frying is not recommended in the first place. Heating refined cooking oils at high temperatures damages the fats and makes them culprits for most digestive system cancers. Re-used cooking oils are dangerous to our health. That is why government agencies arrest people at borders of countries as they attempt to smuggle them. Unfortunately, these agencies cannot come to your home to monitor what kind of cooking oil you are using. The choice is entirely yours. Other bad fats include cheese, butter and most fats that become solid at room temperature. While they may taste great in the mouth, they do a lot of harm in our bodies. On the other hand, good fats as found in olives, avocados and most nuts have the potential to prevent most cancers. We need to eat them in good proportion and regularly, not once in a while as we usually do. Adding avocado in your vegetable salad and some olives, or olive oil spread, is a great idea in fighting cancer. You may also try some other wonderful recipes like having avocado pudding for dessert.

Fats and blood pressure

Unhealthy fats contribute to most cases of high blood pressure in addition to other risk factors like stress, smoking, alcohol, inactivity, obesity, etc. For example if you cook fatty meat, if you let the soup cool, you will discover that it becomes solid. These solid animal fats are also known as cholesterol. These are the fats that kill – these are the fats that form plaques in our blood vessels, thereby raising our blood pressure. You also get a lot of these fats in the so-called high-breed chickens. Sometime I wonder if anybody is supposed to eat those four-to-six week old chickens. But again, the choice is yours. Many people are digging their graves with their own teeth through poor fat choices. In worse scenarios high blood pressure can lead to stroke, heart attack or liver damage. Yet if you choose to eat healthy fats like flax seeds, pumpkin seeds, sunflower seeds, avocado, olives, olive oil and other healthy fats found in whole grains like whole wheat and fresh maize, we can greatly reduce our risk of developing high blood pressure. These good fats do lower the bad fats. That means every time you have wholegrain porridge with some seeds, such as a combination of oats with sunflower seeds or sweet potato and groundnut flour, and sometimes if you are just addicted to the tradition of adding some nuts and seeds when cooking vegetables, you are doing yourself a great favour. In so doing you are reducing your risk of developing chronic conditions.

Just remember when using nut flour, these nuts must be ground the same day you want to use them. The nut flour that was made three weeks ago and was exposed to light may not have the same benefits. Remember the good fats come from the garden.

14. How to Improve Digestion

Do you ever think about what happens to the food you eat? Most of us do not. In most cases we only care about how the food tastes like. We eat anything we like without even thinking how we are going to digest it. Some even eat too much and more often throughout the day. But how does our body handle the food it is given?

First we need to know that digestion starts in the mouth. The time you chew and savour each bite plays a large role in the rest of the digestive process. We don't have teeth in our stomachs, and our intestines cannot do the job that was supposed to be done by your teeth. As the saliva is mixed with food, digestive enzymes begin to break down the food chemicals into smaller units which the body can use. The time you spend chewing your food is important in two ways. Firstly, the food mixing with saliva is important if digestion is to continue properly in the stomach and intestines. But the most important part of it is the time you spend chewing and enjoying each bite as it determines how much satisfaction you get from your meal. It is easy to avoid overeating if you spend enough time chewing your food.

While we may choose to ignore what happens to food after it enters our mouth, oesophagus, stomach and intestines, nevertheless our digestive tract has a complicated process to perform. Taking care of our digestive system is a key to good health. The digestive system is made up of the gastrointestinal (GI) tract plus the liver, pancreas, and gallbladder. The GI tract is a series of hollow organs joined in a long, twisting tube from the mouth to the anus. The hollow organs that make up the GI tract are the mouth, oesophagus, stomach, small intestine, and large intestine which includes the rectum and anus. Food enters the mouth and passes to the anus through the hollow organs of the GI tract. The liver, pancreas, and gallbladder are the solid organs of the digestive system. The digestive system helps the body digest food and make the nutrients available for absorption. We can aid the work of digestion in many ways. Here are some specific suggestions to consider:

No drinking with meals

Drinking liquids at meals dilutes the digestive juices, therefore, it is best to drink (preferably water) at least an hour after a meal or up to half an hour preceding it. Six to eight glasses of water per day is ideal. Fresh, healthy juices are best taken on their own.

Fewer foods per meal

Too large a variety of foods at each meal, which is common in our society, creates an excessive workload for the system. Especially in parties and potlucks people usually struggle with temperance when it comes to variety of foods. Many people today have trained their palates to desire rich, sweet, fatty, spicy foods and are totally unware that simple natural flavours can be enjoyed. In short, our taste buds have been perverted. But this is a habitual pattern we can choose to change. Remember we can train our taste buds to start enjoying and appreciating new flavours in just about 21 days.

Meal times

One of the habits most stressful to the digestive system is eating at the wrong time. Good digestion is not just a matter of what you eat, but when you eat. The digestive tract functions best when given five to six hours to complete its work of digesting each meal before more food is taken into the system. With frequent snacking, such as every two hours, orderly digestive processes may never reach completion. Food which is not properly processed can actually "rot" or ferment in the stomach. In view of such eating patterns, it is easy to see why many people today complain of so much indigestion. Eating most of the food in the evening, particularly late in the evening, is also harmful. The digestive tract was meant to rest during sleeping hours. Considering many people eat a large evening meal followed by dessert and later by a bedtime snack it's a recipe for disaster; it is no wonder many wake up the next day feeling very tired. They awaken unrefreshed, with little ambition beyond a strong desire to stay in bed. After a late evening meal or snack, many have no desire to eat breakfast in the morning. The old adage, "breakfast like a king, lunch like a queen, supper like a pauper", if followed, would be appreciated by the digestive tract. Many have found they function better on two meals in a day. However, the meals referred to are not lunch and supper, but rather breakfast and lunch. Some can adjust to breakfast at 7am, lunch at 1pm, and – nothing to eat until the next day and not even feel hungry. For others, eating breakfast at 8am and lunch at 2pm makes the adjustments easier.

The next time you put food into your mouth, remember what your digestive tract must do to process it. Treat your whole body well and you will feel better and live longer too.

15. Grow Your Own Food

The food you eat can contribute to your health or sickness. Ever wondered that people are more careful on what kind of food they give to their chickens and cows but somehow they do not seem to mind what kind of food to put into their bodies. Some even treat their stomach as if it is a dust bin for all the junk food in town. Remember you are what you eat, and what you eat matters a lot to your mental and physical wellness. One of the secrets to achieve this is to grow your own food organically. This can be done as a backyard kitchen garden or growing some vegetable and medicinal plants in pots and buckets. If you have a large piece of land you can do even more by growing some staple crops like maize, etc. Growing your own food organically enables you and your family to obtain optimum nutrition without the need for expensive and sometimes useless supplements. Yes there are times in clinical practice where good vitamins and minerals supplementation can be necessary and even critical. But if we give our bodies a good foundation of good food from our home garden, we may prevent such times.

Relying on other people to produce our most basic need (food) leaves us terribly vulnerable health wise. The man with a small piece of land which he owns and on which he relies for his food must learn to love that land and care for it wisely. He must respect

God's mighty creation. Health and happiness is the result of living in harmony with God's natural law. Food grown with chemicals like fertilisers and pesticides is better than starving but it is not the best when it comes to nutrition and wellness. I always feel sad when I see people who have a reasonable piece of land surrounding their home covered with concrete and some gorgeous paving to impress visitors. Be kind to yourself – use that piece for an organic home garden. Even worse, some will waste money and energy growing things which nobody will eat like a huge lawn of grass surrounding the home. You do not need a huge piece of land to start growing your own fruits, vegetables and grains. Remember small is beautiful. Yes, there will be other food items that we will always need to buy from the markets. But it is always prudent to grow most of the food we eat, organically. The old Greek physician named Hippocrates said, "Let food be your medicine; and let medicine be your food." Our good health requires a balanced diet which consists of the essential nutrients in correct proportions and comes easily from natural foods. To be a successful food gardener, you will also need to understand your own health and that of your plants. Your needs and their needs must be met.

Modern medical research shows us that whole grains, nuts, seeds, fruits and vegetables protect us from coughs and colds and other infections. They also do protect us against the onset of many cancers. They prevent the thickening of arteries, a major cause of heart disease; they help prevent Alzheimer's, diabetes, anaemia, constipation, and so many other diseases. Take a conscious decision to take your own health, and the health of those closest to you, into your own hands.

PART III
LIFESTYLE DISEASES

16. Tips for Avoiding Diabetes

We all love to hear stories of the old good days. Did you know that there was a time when we didn't know much about diabetes? Not because we were less educated, but the disease was not a pandemic like it is today. Those were the good old days. It was until early in the 1990s that this chronic disease of lifestyle started making headlines in the health centres of the developing countries and today diabetes is like a brand name for most families, especially those living in urban areas. The common symptoms of diabetes are excessive thirst, loss of feeling, general body weakness, excessive hunger, poor eye sight, slow healing of wounds and, in some cases, weight loss. Left uncontrolled, diabetes can lead to blindness, kidney damage, immune disorder, leg amputation, stroke, heart disease and finally, death. The risk factors include diet, a sedentary lifestyle, smoking, alcohol and genetic weakness.

There are two common types of diabetes known as type 1 and type 2. Let us leave the type 1 diabetes topic for now. Type 2 affects 90 percent of diabetic patients and that is what we want to discuss at this point. Many people have blamed genetics, however, that is only the tip of the iceberg. Genetic weaknesses are like a loaded rifle, it is lifestyle that pulls the trigger. Just because you were born with a genetic weakness, inherited from your parents, does not mean that you will one day become diabetic. You need to expose this weakness to a diet and lifestyle that trigger diabetes. The good and comforting news is that diabetes type 2 is potentially preventable whether you were born with the weakness or not.

The dietary factor

If you want to prevent diabetes you need to watch what you eat. In fact, you need to know what the right fuel for your body is. Is it not strange that most people who own cars know exactly what kind of fuel to put in their vehicles while at the same time being ignorant of their body's perfect fuel. You will see a car owner parking at a gas station demanding unleaded petrol for his BMW while at the same time you see him buying junk food (body fuel) to eat from the same gas station shop and expect his body to go a long way. When it comes to diet, many people treat the body like a dustbin. They throw everything down into it as long as it tastes great on the tongue without considering what the food will do in their bodies.

In a nutshell, your body uses food the same way cars use diesel or petrol. Food is our primary source of energy. The moment you start chewing your food, digestion begins. We start digesting carbohydrates in our mouth with the enzymes found in our saliva. By the time the food items reach the second half of our small intestine the original food you ate is completely broken down into glucose, amino acids, fat acids, vitamins and minerals, assuming that your digestive system is in perfect state. All the nutrients, including the glucose (the body's major fuel), are absorbed into the blood stream. Through the power of the hormone insulin, glucose is injected into your cells where it is burned as energy similar to what an engine of a car does.

Eat whole foods

One thing that I have learnt in life as a Clinical Nutritionist is that we cannot improve the food God created for us. If we eat food closer to its natural state as it came from the hands of our benevolent Creator, without much refining, it will be a big step in preventing diabetes. The way we eat fresh maize is how God intended that we should eat the grains. Nothing should be lost from the grain. If you want to eat rice, wheat products, barley, or maize products, always demand the wholegrain products. Whether it is bread or pasta, it must come from the whole grain. The outer layer of the grain (bran), which is usually thrown away when the grain is refined, is rich in functional carbohydrate known as fibre. Fibre absorbs excess glucose, thereby preventing diabetes. Many people think that whole foods are for those who are diabetic, that is true, but remember they are the best foods for those who are not diabetic today so that they do not become diabetic tomorrow. Adding legumes, fresh vegetables and whole fruits to a wholegrain diet is the way to go if we are interested in avoiding diabetes. Refined food is one of the triggers of diabetes type 2 – you eat this food at your own risk.

Exercise is critical to a total lifestyle that prevents and even manage diabetes. It helps to burn glucose and manages your body weight which is one of the key factors in preventing diabetes. Remember, weight management does not mean becoming thin so that you can wear size zero kinds of dresses. It is about regaining your normal weight in proportion to your height, usually known as Body Mass Index (BMI). To achieve that, exercise must be part of your whole, healthy lifestyle including diet, rest and stress management. Brisk walking is the best, so are some other aerobic exercises. Your fitness program must be scheduled throughout the week as a priority, and not "bumped" for seemingly more important items. Yes, it is possible to prevent diabetes.

17. Walk Out of Obesity

Some years ago people were confusing being overweight with good health. Gaining weight was a symbol of status and sometimes an indication that someone was healthy. Yes, there was a time being overweight was considered a sign of success. We may all remember times when our friends congratulated us for gaining weight. Today, we know that being overweight and obesity increase the likelihood of a number of chronic diseases and other health problems. Obesity is a medical condition in which excess body fat has accumulated to the extent that it may have an adverse effect on health, leading to reduced life expectancy and/or increased health problems.

Being overweight and obesity carry an extremely high risk for diabetes, hypertension, heart diseases, stroke, gall bladder diseases, back pain, heart failure, varicose veins, menstrual abnormalities, etc.

Why are we getting so big?

Some have blamed genetics; this may be true. But only in rare cases. Diet and lifestyle are the major contributing factors in weight gain. Eating a diet high in refined and processed foods; e.g. cakes, biscuits, white bread, fried foods, fatty foods and most fast food products available in our supermarkets today, is one of the culprits of weight gain.

If we are not physically active, we are most likely to gain weight and we may become obese. The good news is that being overweight and obesity are reversible simply by going back to the basics of good nutrition and physical activity. Other factors like stress and rest need also be taken into consideration.

What shall I eat to lose weight?

Do not go on a diet but rather adopt a healthier dietary lifestyle. It must be a way of life, not an event. Make sure you are eating whole grains instead of refined ones. Whole grains are high in fibre which assist in binding excess fat in the digestive tract and make it part of the excrement. Fibre also binds excess glucose which may end up converted into fats anyway. Other sources of fibre include legumes like beans, pigeon peas, peas, chick peas, lentils, cow peas, etc. Every time we eat natural fruits and vegetables we give ourselves a cocktail packed with vitamins and minerals which help to detox the fat in our bodies. Fruits and vegetables do contain some fibre as well. Taking fruits such as lemons, apples, pineapples, oranges and grapes are excellent choices. Dark green vegetables like spinach, pumpkin leaves, and indigenous vegetables with some salads, from time to time, is a great idea.

Walk out your weight

Walking has been the best exercise as far as losing weight is concerned. Other forms of exercise may also be commendable. Vigorous exercises may not be good for beginners, always start with gentle exercise and increase the intensity with time. I have met people who go around jogging every morning trying to lose some kilos without much success. Brisk walking is the best as it encourages more intake of oxygen through deep breathing. The more oxygen you breathe in the more fat you burn. Running on the other hand makes you fail to breathe normally, hence less intake of oxygen. Gentle cycling is just as good, so are other gentle aerobics. The time that you go for a walk also matters. We burn more fats if we go for a walk early in the morning before breakfast – but make sure you have a glass or two of pure water before going for a walk. Warm water is much better than cold water. Just get up and do it, you will soon wonder why you never did it before.

18. The Heart Under Attack

I remember the first time I saw someone dying of a heart attack eight years ago; it was hard to believe that our friend was dead in just a few seconds. Hundreds of thousands of people die every year from heart attacks worldwide. A heart attack is like a sudden explosion. Technically, a heart attack occurs when the supply of nutrient-rich blood to the heart muscle is reduced or stopped. If the blood supply is shut down for a long time, muscle cells die from lack of oxygen. If enough cells die, the victim will also die. Sometimes, if only a small part of the heart muscle is deprived of oxygen, the victim can recover. Heart attacks are frightening for both the victim and for the victim's companions.

One does not need to be a fanatic in order to admit that modern, civilized man is living somewhat dangerously. Just think of all the conveniences we have gained from technology in our age of motor cars and mechanization. They bring with them less activity outdoors. Our indulgence in refined and fatty food products does not exactly contribute to healthy hearts either. The arteries degenerate as a result of the drawbacks of our lifestyle, symptoms of heart problems appear much too early and sometimes bring an early end to our lives. Even the World Health Organization has pointed out that an unhealthy diet, sedentary lifestyle, excessive smoking and heavy drinking of alcohol are the major culprits of heart attacks.

Dinner that kills

Not everything that we eat will cause a heart attack. Some foods may help to prevent it. The main culprits are excessive amounts of fat and cholesterol. These fats may cause narrowing, hardening, and eventually plugging up of vital arteries that supply the heart with oxygen. The process is known in medical terms as atherosclerosis. Human beings are born with clean, flexible arteries. They should stay that way for life. Excessive intake of animal-based foods, which are high in cholesterol and dip fried foods, even foods with too much salt, is like digging your own grave with your teeth. On the other hand, whole grains, nuts, legumes, fruits and vegetables do prevent heart attacks and they can keep your heart young at any age. In cultures where people eat a balanced diet mainly from whole plant-based foods, high in fibre, heart attacks are almost non-existent.

Smoking and alcohol

Scientists have proven that smoking doubles your risk of having a heart attack and doubles, triples, or quadruples your risk of sudden cardiac death. So, do not smoke. The sooner you quit, the sooner your risk will start to decline. Former smokers can completely lower their risk of sudden cardiac death within ten years of quitting. If the alcohol content is excessive in your blood, your heart will be in danger. If a lot of alcohol is flowing in your blood stream, the nutrient and oxygen-rich blood is less able to nourish the heart.

19. Alcohol and Cancer Prevention

If you have seen someone slowly dying in agony from cancer you will agree with me that cancer is an evil worth preventing where and when we can. There are many risk factors that may contribute and promote the growth of cancer cells in our bodies. They include diet, stress, hormones, environmental toxins, genetic weakness, occupation, smoking, alcohol and other unhealthy practices like a sedentary lifestyle, etc.

Alcohol feeds cancer

However, in this topic we would like to focus on the link between alcohol and cancer. It is now common knowledge that alcohol intake can promote and encourage the growth of cancer cells. Alcohol is associated with an increased risk of a number of cancers. Breast cancer in women is linked to alcohol intake. Taking alcoholic drinks also increases the risk of cancers of the mouth, oesophagus, pharynx and larynx, colorectal cancer, liver cancer, stomach and ovaries. If you have cancer cells, for whatever reason, alcohol promotes the growth of these cancer cells, it is like applying fertilizer in a weed garden. While it is true that not everyone who drinks will develop cancer, on the whole, medical scientists have found that some cancers are more common in people who drink more alcohol than others. It is not just people who drink very heavily who have higher risks. Regularly drinking a pint of premium lager or a large glass of wine a day or less can increase the risk of mouth, throat, oesophageal (foodpipe), breast and bowel cancers.

Modern day syndrome

It is sad today to see a lot of young people indulging in alcoholic drinks. If this trend continues, we are not going to win the war against cancer. Our dream to conquer cancer as a people will turn into an endless nightmare. Another sad development today is that of young and old women who are confusing the drinking habit with civilization. Some years ago drinking alcohol was considered a hobby of some men. It was rare to see a woman drinking alcohol and, on average, our women used to live longer than men. But today we see an increase in the number of women who are taking alcoholic drinks, branding themselves as social drinkers. Peer pressure is forcing a number of young ladies, especially in corporate circles today, to start drinking. Kitchen parties and bridal showers have become modern alcohol drinking pubs for most women. Medical researchers are telling us that women can hardly tolerate alcohol due to hormonal issues, even a little alcoholic drink taken on a regular basis can place a woman at risk of developing cancer much faster than a man. It is a strange thing that if something tastes bad and bitter or burns on the tongue, once one has become used to it, the palate even comes to like it. But should not exactly this reaction move us to embrace only good and healthy habits? Of course it should! And by the way, the craving to drink something can be satisfied in a completely harmless way. There are many healthy and delicious non-alcoholic drinks out there and, even better, you can make your own healthy drinks at home like fruit juices of your choice in season. It is certainly unwise to expose oneself to the danger of cancer because of some so-called societal pressure.

Heavy drinkers

The more alcohol you drink, the higher the risk of developing cancer and other diseases. Heavy drinking can cause cirrhosis of the liver, which can, in turn, cause liver cancer. Heavy drinking can also lead to stroke, high blood pressure, pancreatitis and injuries. Most men who are diagnosed with liver cancer in our hospitals are heavy drinkers. The liver is one of the delicate organs you cannot live without. We only have one liver in a lifetime, when it is gone that is the end of life. Drinking a lot of alcohol increases the risk of cancer, whether you drink it at a go during weekends or a bit at a time.

It is easy, change your lifestyle

Do yourself a favour, dying from cancer is a very painful way of dying. While all of us can get cancer due to various risk factors, we should not deliberately invite this plague through the drinking of alcohol, smoking, bad diet, or unhealthy lifestyle practices. Change the way you socialize, spend quality time with your children, play with them, be a parent to them; as a father or mother your kids need you more now than when they will be grown-ups. Enjoy some hobbies like cooking and baking or start a walking club instead of attending ladies' parties every weekend. Young people, avoid bad company, join a social fitness group, become a member of a prayer band at your church or join a singing group and find better ways of spending your leisure time.

20. Building Better Joints – Arthritis

Arthritis is a general term commonly used to describe diseases in the joints. The word just means "inflammation of a joint." Our joints allow us to move. They are the "hinges" of the body. They need to be well lubricated, strong and healthy. Just like the ligaments and muscles, joints wear with use and need to be constantly repaired, a process that normally occurs during sleep. How does a joint tell you when it is getting damaged? It begins to hurt and may get stiff. It may also swell up and become red. Often people with the disease feel worse in the mornings and the pain and stiffness lessen as the joint is warmed. All these signs may be common to most forms of arthritis.

There are many different types of arthritis. The most common is osteoarthritis. Osteoarthritis usually occurs when a joint's blood supply becomes inadequate for its needed functions. Just as a heart will weaken and ultimately fail when the coronary arteries clog up with plaque, so joints begin to break down when the arteries supplying them become narrowed or obstructed. Gradually ligaments weaken, joint fluids decrease, and cartilage wears away.

Weight-bearing joints, such as the ones in the spine, knees, and hips, are commonly affected. This is worsened by extra body weight. Just as a bridge has a load limit, so do the joints. Osteoarthritis can also occur at any time after an injury or excessive wear-and-tear to a joint, as often happen in sport. Many people believe that osteoarthritis is the most common cause of backache. This is not so. In fact, only about 10 percent of backaches are caused by osteoarthritis or disc problems. Up to 80 percent of lower back pain sufferers are victims of either overworked or under-exercised muscles. A strained muscle may suddenly go into a spasm and become a painful, knotty mass. Once serious back injury has been ruled out, the important thing to do with backaches is to get on your feet and start walking. Back specialists say that prolonged bed rest will do more harm than good, because rest causes your back muscles to weaken rapidly. Fortunately most back problems resolve themselves in four to 12 weeks.

Preventing arthritis

Here are some tips to prevent arthritis. Keep your weight down – that is the biggest favour you can do for your back. Avoid high heels (over one inch). They tilt the pelvis and throw the back out of alignment. Strengthen your back and abdominal muscles with stretching exercises. Walk, swim or cycle at least twenty minutes, five times a week. Eat a diet low in fat and high in fibre. These measures are important for back pain as well as for all kinds of arthritis. Gout is another type of arthritis. From antiquity this disease has been associated with the lifestyles of the rich people who eat too much rich food and have too little activity. Even the poor who are taking alcoholic drinks and animal products can also be victims of gout.

A largely plant-based diet, which is low in fat and high in fibre, has been shown to improve circulation to the joints. In time, this kind of diet may help open up some of the narrowed arteries. Fat thickens the blood and slows down its circulation. Fat also causes red blood cells to stick to each other, so that they are unable to navigate the smaller arterioles to deliver needed oxygen. The wise man summed it up well: "Pleasant words are a honeycomb, sweet to the soul and healing to the bones." Proverbs 16:24. Fight for your health. Stay active. Most people who get better are the ones who take an active role in bringing about positive, permanent changes in their lifestyles. It is never too late to start.

21. Osteoporosis

Protecting Your Bones

Today osteoporosis is silently and painlessly weakening the bones of millions of unsuspecting people. Worldwide, one out of every three women over the age of 50 is suffering from osteoporosis. Though commonly viewed as a disease of older women, 20 percent of its victims are men. The statistics may differ from country to country depending on the population general lifestyle.

Just what is osteoporosis?

It is a disease of the bones. Strong bones gradually become thin and brittle, their insides soft and spongy. As a result, these bones can break easily. Whether it is a wrist, spine, or hip, fractures due to osteoporosis can significantly decrease one's quality of life.

Statistics show that this disease is steadily rising around the world. According to the World Health Organization, the number of hip fractures worldwide, due to osteoporosis, is expected to increase 300 percent by the mid-21st century. Only one out of three people who break a hip regain their independence. One out of four die during the first year after their fracture and nearly half of those who survive still cannot walk without aid.

So how does osteoporosis develop?

Bones increase in strength and thickness especially during childhood and early teen years. After that, bone strength continues to develop at a slower rate until around age 35. At this stage the process gradually reverses itself, and small amounts of bone are lost each year. This bone loss worsens in women after menopause. When certain harmful lifestyle habits are present, this loss occurs more rapidly, greatly increasing your risk of getting osteoporosis. Day by day, many people are unconsciously making withdrawals from their bone reserves. How does this occur? Research has identified many bone-robbing lifestyle factors; here are a few of them – cigarettes and alcohol disrupt the body's calcium balance in many ways, from the formation of healthy bone cells to hindering necessary calcium absorption. Using caffeinated beverages, such as coffee, tea, and soft drinks increases the loss of calcium through the kidneys. Not getting enough exercise is an especially important risk factor in today's modern society. Our bones cannot thicken and grow stronger without regular, weight-bearing exercise, such as walking. To retain their minerals, bones need to be pressed, pushed, pulled, and twisted by exercise.

Consuming too much phosphorous, especially found in meat, dairy products, and certain soft drinks as well as too much salt in the diet will bind up calcium, pulling it out of the body as these substances are excreted by the kidneys. All of these things can slowly rob calcium from your bones and increase your risk of osteoporosis. Other natural foods like pumpkin leaves, sweet potato leaves, black jack leaves, broccoli, cauliflower, spinach, beetroot, carrots and seeds like sunflower may assist in preventing the loss of bone mass. Some villagers in African countries, especially women, live up to the age of 90 years without osteoporosis. It is ascribed to their simple village diet of local fruit and vegetables which are good for calcium balance. The active rural life is another blessing for these women. Without knowing it, they do prevent osteoporosis in their lifetime.

How can you tell if you have osteoporosis?

Without professional help, you cannot, not until you fracture a bone or start shrinking in height, and that is quite late in the disease. You should be tested if you are middle-aged or older and have a lifestyle that predisposes you to get this disease. In conclusion, we have seen that osteoporosis is becoming an epidemic in many countries throughout the world. Yet, you need not be one of its victims. A good diet and an active, healthy lifestyle will go a long way to help keep your bones in the best of shape! Remember, your bone bank is like your regular bank account. If you deposit more than you withdraw, your balance grows. On the other hand, when calcium is robbed from the bones, the balance diminishes, putting you at risk of developing osteoporosis.

Our Heavenly Father stands ready to bless all who desire and make an effort to live healthfully. Why not ask Him for wisdom and help to make the necessary changes? In Isaiah we are promised, "The Lord will guide you continually, and satisfy your soul in drought, and **strengthen your bones**; you shall be like a watered garden, and like a spring of water, whose waters do not fail." (Isaiah 58:11).

22. Reclaiming Your Lost Immunity

What do the common colds, asthma, and cancer have in common? They are the result of a breakdown in the body's defence system. Let us take a closer look at the immune system, the army within our body. The immune system is equipped with legions of mobile soldiers, with an arsenal of deadly weapons and a sophisticated chemical communication network. These defenders must be on duty every minute of every day in order to detect and destroy the enemy. Even one surviving germ or cancer cell can be potentially life threatening. One out of every 100 cells belongs to the body's armed forces, an army totalling nearly one trillion white blood cells! Here are some of the many functions of these Special Forces.

Phagocytes are the army's foot soldiers. They are the first ones to arrive on the battlefield. They engulf invading germs and dissolve the enemy with powerful enzymes. Lymphocytes perform other important tasks. Some carry weapons that destroy cells infected with invading viruses. Other lymphocytes target cancer cells, while others produce highly specialised weapons called antibodies. While the immune system is designed to protect the body from diseases, if it malfunctions it is also capable of causing diseases. Allergic disorders such as asthma and hay fever occur when the immune system mistakenly battles against normally harmless substances such as house dust, pollens, and certain foods. Histamine, one of the chemicals released in the process, is responsible for some of the typical symptoms of allergies like itching, runny nose and watery eyes.

In diseases such as rheumatoid arthritis and childhood onset diabetes (Type 1) the immune system attacks and destroys the body's own tissues. That is why these are called autoimmune diseases. A strong, healthy immune system has mechanisms that prevent disorders like these before they begin. AIDS is probably one of the most devastating diseases of the immune system. An enemy virus invades and debilitates the body's immune system, so that its forces are weakened and overcome by infections and cancer.

How can we strengthen our immune system?

Fortunately, there are numerous ways we can build up our immune system. For example: clean, fresh outdoor air can actually inhibit cancer growth and help correct allergic disorders such as asthma and hay fever. Fresh air also aids in protecting the immune forces from the devastating effects of stress. Polluted air is a major health concern worldwide, and asthmatics are very sensitive to pollutants. With diminishing air quality, it is not surprising that asthma is increasing at an alarming rate. Pure water is another vital ingredient for healthy immune function. Water is a potent detoxifying agent, flushing germs and other pollutants out of the body. The bloodstream, which is the highway to transport the immune system's troops, is kept flowing freely by adequate amounts of water. In addition, the mucus membranes of the nose and mouth also need plenty of water to maintain a protective barrier against invading germs.

Exercise makes the circulatory system stronger; this includes the lungs, heart and blood vessels. With regular physical activity, the bloodstream can transport troops to the front lines with greater efficiency. Exercise also neutralises the harmful effects of stress by stimulating the release of natural "feel good" chemicals like endorphins. Stress is especially counteracted when exercise is combined with the immune system's allies like fresh air and sunlight. Rest plays an important role in immune function. The hours of deep sleep before midnight are prime time for the repair and replacement of worn out cells and tissues. During this period, the body's housekeepers and mechanics work best to restore its guardians to top fighting shape. Under ideal sleep conditions, the casualties that occur are more rapidly replaced by new white blood cells.

When regular sleep hours are disturbed, there is a price to pay. In today's world irregular work schedules disrupt sleeping and eating patterns and compromise the immune system's performance. It is not surprising that irregular working hours are associated with a greater risk of colds and flu, serious illnesses and even a shortened life expectancy. By eating natural foods that contain an abundance of vitamins and minerals, you can help keep your immune system operating smoothly. Vitamins A, C, and E along with the minerals zinc and magnesium, are in special demand. Fortunately, an abundance of these nutrients are available by eating a variety of fresh fruit, vegetables, whole grains and nuts.

For a healthy immune system, the body needs certain essential fats. The body cannot manufacture these, so they must be obtained from nutritious food. One class of friendly fats is the omega-3 fatty acids, which empowers the cancer-killing forces and inhibit cancer cell growth. Flax seed, walnuts, green soybeans and spinach are all good sources of omega-3 fats. On the other hand, diets including the regular use of processed or refined fats and oils disable the cancer-fighting forces and promote the growth and spread of cancer cells. These should be avoided. What about sugar? Refined sugar, like refined fats, is an enemy of the immune system. Sugar quickly deactivates the germ-killing foot soldiers – the phagocytes. For example, just one soft drink, containing 12 teaspoons of sugar, is enough to weaken the protective ability of our body's white blood cells by 60 percent, for five hours. Alcohol, tobacco and caffeine are all detrimental to the body's defences. Make good choices and keep your immune system strong.

PART IV
LIVE WELL

23. Exercise – for the Health of It

Did you know that simply getting off the couch and walking for 30 to 40 minutes, three to five times a week, can reduce our risk of premature death from cancer, high blood pressure and diabetes by 20 to 40 percent? Ever wonder why we hear about people in other parts of the world who live longer and active lives. We read about people in Northern China who live up to 145 years and they are not in old age homes yet. The valley of Hunza in Pakistan has a number of its citizens who have celebrated their 100th happy birthdays. There must be a number of wellness pillars that have contributed to such quality of life in those communities and one of it is physical activity.

Physical exercise is the law of health. This principle goes right back to the Garden of Eden. The original paradise was indeed a beautiful, tranquil place. But contrary to some stereotypes, Adam and Eve did not lie all day on a riverbank in Eden, drinking fresh coconut juice. They did not just lounge around looking at flowers and birds. While the Creator could have designed their lives to be quite labour-free and passive, He had something else in mind. "The Lord God took the man and put him in the Garden of Eden to work it and take care of it" (Genesis 2:15). Paradise, for Adam and Eve, was not a world of idleness. Eden did not automatically meet all their needs. They were responsible for cultivating the garden. It was God's way of keeping them physically active.

It is exercise that brings in the nutrients via the bloodstream to your muscles, your bones, and your joints. That means even a good diet without exercise may not give you the expected health miracle. I remember our good old days in Africa where life was full of activity. We had to grow our own vegetables, schools were far from homes and we had to do a lot of walking to get there and people were not ashamed to look dirty due to some kind of handwork. Even making food was not such a simple task as firewood was sought from a distance. Manual work was the order of the day and rarely did we hear about cancer, diabetes, heart attack or stroke in those days.

Today, we are living a life in the fast lane. Everything is across the street. There is no sweating. We ride cars, use public transport and we do soft jobs. We even associate walking with poverty. For most of us, walking is for the poor or the less blessed.

Exercise helps get the oxygen through your blood system. This helps in growing, mending, promoting, and maintaining your body. When you take in your car for a tune-up, it really runs better. Then after a while, it needs another tune-up. The body operates in pretty much the same way. Activity is the way we tune up. Want to feel better, have more energy and perhaps even live longer? Start with exercise. The health benefits of regular exercise and physical activity are difficult to ignore. Just check in our communities today. The less physically active we are, the more cases of chronic conditions exist. Worse still, we see young people taking the path of sedentary lifestyle at an early stage, unlike the old good days when young people used to be engaged in outdoor games. Things like PlayStations and multimedia equipment are the time consumers for the youth. We should do more physical activity than just watching other people doing it on the TV screen while we are busy changing channels using remote controls.

Exercise can help prevent excess weight gain or help maintain weight loss. When you engage in physical activity, you burn calories. The more intense the activity, the more calories you burn. Gone are the days when we used to confuse weight gain with good health or as a symbol of wealth. Today we know that being overweight and obesity are signs of illness. You do not need to set aside large chunks of time for exercise to reap weight-loss benefits. If you cannot do an actual workout, get more active throughout the day in simple ways – by taking the stairs instead of the elevator or reviving up your household chores instead of leaving everything to a helper.

In fact, regular physical activity can help you prevent or manage a wide range of health problems and concerns, including stroke, metabolic syndrome, type 2 diabetes, depression, and certain types of cancer, arthritis and falls.

Your mental health will benefit too. After a stressful day a workout at the gym, or a brisk 30-minute walk, can help. Physical activity stimulates various brain chemicals that may leave you feeling happier and more relaxed. You may also feel better about your appearance and yourself when you exercise regularly, you will like what you will see in the mirror which can boost your confidence and improve your self-esteem.

Are you having difficulty sleeping during the night? Doing exercise regularly can help you sleep better and faster. Just do not exercise too close to bedtime, or you may be too energized to fall asleep.

So whether you decide to start walking or join some social sport group, physical activity can be a motivating way to spend some time with family and friends. It gives you a chance to unwind, enjoy the outdoors or simply engage in activities that make you happy. Start a walking club in your community, hit the hiking trails or get into the garden if you have one. Find a physical activity you enjoy, and just do it. If you get bored, try something new.

Remember to check with your doctor before starting a new exercise program if you have a chronic condition like heart disease or any health concerns. And the benefits of exercise are yours for the taking, regardless of your age, sex or physical ability. So just keep moving!

24. Creating a Healthy Environment

Many times when we talk of environment we always think of our cities. But take a moment to reflect about your personal environment both at your home and in your workplace. Are your surroundings cheerful and healthy? Are they places that nurture your soul and recharge your mind? Do you feel calm and happy when you're at your home or work? Do they comfort you, offer you an opportunity for growth, and give you a sense of peace? Many of us don't care much about the choice of a home for our families. God knew the effect our environment would have on us. That's why He placed the first family in the garden.

Though we can't expect to recreate the Garden of Eden, we can take away the lessons from it and then apply them to our own living surroundings, thereby making our homes and our workplaces much healthier. The closer we come to making our personal environments like the original Garden of Eden, the more of its health benefits will we experience. Many of us today do not appreciate nature. That is why you will find most home and office grounds are covered with concrete instead of plants. The plants use carbon dioxide and they give out oxygen while humans use oxygen and give out carbon dioxide. Do we understand why God gave the garden full of vegetation as a home for man?

What constitutes environment?

Our environment encompasses all that is around us. It impacts us through our sight, hearing, smell, touch and taste. Our work and home environment probably impact our health the most because we spend most of our time in them. So paying attention and striving to create a healthy environment in both places give rich rewards.

The home environment

No matter how humble, there is no place like home. You may not have the most expensive furniture imported from overseas. Maybe you have most of your household tools from second hand shops, but still you can create a healthy environment that promotes wellness at home. Make your home a peaceful green spot in contrast to the harshness of the world at large. Create a place that you, your family and guests will be blessed, a place that nurtures and restores everyone who enters. Your home reflects you. Your home should make you feel good; it should recharge and revive the health of all who enter. It should be a place of comfort, peace, and love. Parents as home makers have a responsibility to make our homes the healthiest environment possible. Our children will love to be at home more than any place in the world.

The costs of dirt and clutter

Let us learn to keep our environment clean, organized, and in order. These habits will help promote peace and health. Clutter, mess, and a lack of organization in our home can serve as stressors, or may even be a symptom of stress. Living in a mess can impact our social lives, too, which is very important to our well-being. We might feel that the house is not clean enough to have loved ones over and, therefore, we miss out on the enrichment that socializing with those we love brings. Living in dirty environments can contribute to depression and bad behaviour. Take a moment to notice how you feel next time you walk into a room that is disorganized and messy, and then notice how you feel when you walk into a room that is neat, clean and inviting. It makes a big different wellness wise.

Bring nature inside

We can benefit even more by bringing nature inside. Growing plants whether for food, healing herbs or just flowers indoors aids in removing several toxic chemicals from the air in building interiors. Planting a garden, fruit orchard, or just some beautiful trees surrounding the home or office building can make your health ten times better. Remember human beings get fresh oxygen from the plants. The closer we get to the original environment the healthier we will be.

25. Vacations and Good Health

We all love vacations, but hardly ever take them. Many people think that it's a waste of time and money to go on vacations. Regularly scheduled vacations are a wonderful way to put "life" back into your existence. But the truth is that we become more productive at work or even at home after a vacation. Even better if you make it a family affair, it will also help you to feel closer to the family. It's not a good idea to take some work projects to vacation as this kills the purpose of the holiday. This is time to relax and reflect on what you have achieved and how you can do things better in future while having quality time. The key is to stay healthy during holidays. As we all know holidays come in different shapes and sizes. It is our custom worldwide to celebrate end of the year with parties and celebrations. We cannot avoid celebrating Christmas and happy New Year even if we don't believe in them. If you don't organize one at home, you will be invited to a number of them. For the working class they usually have a few office and business parties before taking off for holidays, only to be welcomed by more parties from family and friends. But how can you stay healthy and lean during the festival seasons and vacations? I remember a friend who had a heart attack after enjoying a dish high in cheese on Christmas. He had hypertension; probably the high cholesterol meal plus the excitement triggered the heart attack. Why does the time for vacation and cerebration somehow give us mental permission to indulge in every junk food that comes in our path?

Wise eating

Whether you are mingling at your annual office party, out on a game drive, or stranded at your in-laws' for an early Christmas visit, you need to exercise the power of choice by eating wisely. While the endless parties offer numerous opportunities to indulge, don't lose your will power and always plan ahead on what you want to eat and what you want to avoid. Keep your enemy food out of your kitchen. Any junk food available within your home, it's easy to devour at exciting moments when there's a lapse of judgment. Even healthy foods can become unhealthy if you eat too much. Wise food choices can help you survive the vacations and holidays with your dignity and your waistline intact.

Wise shopping

When shopping for a vacation or home parties make sure you buy more wholesome foods. Buy more fruits like watermelon, pineapple, apple, mango, papaya, grapes, etc. Depending on your menu, you can make a delicious fruit salad mixed with plain yoghurt or just a fruity platter up for grabs while sharing the old time stories to your grandkids. Get some whole wheat flour which you can use to bake some special times delicacies. Be creative or wander through some good recipe books and you will find something special that you can bake for your family and friends. Think of baking wonderful products like carrot cakes, pumpkin and coconut bread, banana and orange muffins made with real whole food ingredients not just flavors. Remember every time you eat whole foods, you are giving yourself a cocktail of proteins, carbohydrates, vitamins, minerals and antioxidants. You will never go wrong if you bless yourself with some Greek salad, just make sure you add some avocado and olive oil to it. The cucumbers, lettuce, carrots, onion, olives, green pepper are all detox vegetables. For sure you cannot afford to have a party these days without something to drink. Include in your shopping list a wide variety of whole fruit juices. Home-made are the best, especially those fresh fruits in season. These wholesome juices are many times better than alcoholic and fizzy drinks. Unwise shopping and eating can turn what was supposed to be a time of cerebration into an endless nightmare.

Balance pleasure and rest

If you snooze you lose, that's the usual slogan during celebration times. Maybe it's because most fun events are organized during the night. However, if you sacrifice sleep for a number of days know that you are doing that at the cost of your health. It's important to know when to say goodbye or when to walk away. Aim to have seven to eight hours of interrupted sleep if your vacations are to be a blessing.

A good sleep helps the whole system to recover and prepares you for the joys of the next day. Depriving yourself from sleep in the name of happy times is not a good idea. When the holidays are over you will suffer from fatigue and instead of enjoying your work, you will need another holiday to recover. Organize some activities which will require more burning of calories. Think of activities like swimming, hiking, cycling or just some nature walk.

Live a life of praise

Above all, remember to thank our benevolent creator for His mercies and kindness for the year gone. The gift of life, the food we eat, the humble homes where we live, are all blessings from God. Living a life of praise and counting your blessings is one of the therapies for overcoming stress. Focus on the sunny side of life. Remember even among thorns there are roses growing.

26. Kill Stress, Before it Kills You

Stress has been linked with almost every medical problem we have like heart attacks, strokes, hypertension, ulcers, colitis, asthma, arthritis, even cancer. It can invite other problems like low job performance, fatigue, boredom, restlessness and depression. Stress occurs in any situation that requires making a change. That's why even an event like getting married can be stressful. Most people define stress by problems that confront them and concerns they have to deal with.

Little stress can be beneficial; it can improve our awareness, promote alertness and result in a wonderful performance. The positive stress which comes as a result of something good happening or achieved can produce feelings of extreme pleasure. Some examples might be winning a competition, receiving a job promotion, praise from a co-worker or a child's good school report. Then there's stress that exhausts and depresses, for example: a job loss, legal problems, rebellious children, divorce, the death of a loved one, etc. Health is the ability to adapt to life's stresses. Some stressful situations in life are unavoidable, but it matters to our health how we handle these situations. We live in stressful times and stress, if left uncontrolled, can kill.

Some people hardly seem to be affected by stressors (outside stress triggers). They maintain a sense of perspective and a sense of humour. They remain calm in the midst of adversity and catastrophe. Other people are overwhelmed by a lesser number of stressors and slide downhill quickly, losing relationships, jobs, and eventually their mental and physical health. It may seem that there's nothing you can do about stress. The bills won't stop coming, there will never be more hours in a day, and your career and family responsibilities will always be demanding. But you have more control than you might think. In fact, the simple realization that you're in control of your life is the foundation of stress management. Managing stress is all about taking charge of your thoughts, emotions, schedule, the way you deal with problems and trusting in God who is greater than our problems and bigger than our confusion. The knowledge that your Creator has a better plan for your life, will keep you going even when the going gets tough.

Stress management starts with identifying the sources of stress in your life. This isn't as easy as it sounds. Your true sources of stress aren't always obvious, and it's all too easy to overlook your own stress-inducing thoughts, feelings, and behaviors by blaming others for the negative things happening in our lives. Sure, you may know that you're constantly worried about work deadlines. But maybe it's your procrastination, rather than the actual job demands, that leads to deadline stress. To identify your true sources of stress, look closely at your habits, attitude and excuses. Until you accept responsibility for the role you play in creating or maintaining it, your stress level will remain outside your control. Choose good thoughts and avoid dwelling on negatives. Our minds were created with the power to choose what kind of things we should think about. When the day is over count your blessings not your sorrows, count your friends not your enemies, share the good things that happened during the day. "A merry heart works as good as medicine." – Proverbs 17:22.

Not all stress can be avoided, and it's not healthy to avoid a situation that needs to be addressed. You may be surprised, however, by the number of stressors in your life that you can eliminate when you identify them. Some sources of stress are unavoidable. You can't prevent or change stressors such as the death of a loved one, a serious illness, or a national recession. In such cases, the best way to cope with stress is to accept things as they are. Acceptance may be difficult, but in the long run, it's easier than railing against a situation you can't change. Don't try to control the uncontrollable. Many things in life are beyond our control particularly the behaviour of other people. Rather than stressing out over them, focus on the things you can control such as the way you choose to react to their behaviour. When facing major challenges, try to look at them as opportunities for personal growth. If your own poor choices contributed to a stressful situation, reflect on them and learn from your mistakes. Share your feelings. Talk to a trusted friend or make an appointment with a therapist. Expressing what you're going through can be very healing, even if there's nothing you can do to alter the stressful situation. Learn to forgive. Accept the fact that we live in an imperfect world and that people make mistakes. Let go of anger and resentment. Free yourself from negative energy by forgiving and moving on. Connect with others. Spend time with positive people who enhance your life. A strong support system will buffer you from the negative effects of stress. Do something you enjoy every day. Make time for leisure activities that bring you joy, whether it be sawing, playing the piano, or working in your garden. Keep your sense of humour. This includes the ability to laugh at yourself. The act of laughing helps your body fight stress in a number of ways. Above all things Trust in God. Nothing is comforting in trying times like faith and hope in a loving God. I have seen many people who have survived stressful times because of their trust in God.

PART V
SOCIAL WELLNESS

27. Social Wellness

Ever wonder that some people who seem to have less income and material wealth are sometimes the healthiest and the happiest. I remember reading a story of men in the valley of Hunza in Pakistan. The guys are poor by all economic standards yet the men never stop smiling. From their faces you can sense genuine happiness. This does not suggest that we must be poor. I believe it is prudent to be ambitious and invest intelligently for the future. But in these days of love of materialism, when we hear more prayers of financial breakthroughs than prayers for salvation, we are not winning the war on poor health. Another missing ingredient in our medicine box is social wellness. People are naturally social beings. The quality of our social life equals the quality of our health.

Family social health

Did you know that even couples who are happily married have stronger immune systems than their single peers or even worse, those in miserable relationships? Of course marriage is a double edged sword. A happy marriage is a source of good health. If you are blessed with a wonderful family thank God, it works just as well as medicine. Every time you smile from your heart, the production of your white blood cells increases, that means a powerful resistance to illness. The sense of security in a trusting relationship also does the trick in boosting general health. On the other hand a toxic marriage, if nothing is done to it, can destroy your health and reduce you to a chronic patient. You start with mental breakdown due to depression. When mental health is under attack, the whole body system sympathises. Mental breakdown can lead to ulcers, cancers, blood pressure and other side effects which may include overeating or undereating. Hence, it is important to do whatever it takes to build a happy family. Yes challenges will come, electricity and water bills will never stop coming, the kids' school fees still need to be paid, but do not allow these day to day issues to steal the happiness which money cannot buy. Take more time to chat and play together. If you have kids, spare some quality time every day to chat to them. Their stories may not make sense to you but your company is therapeutic to them. Children who feel loved by parents do perform better in school in addition to developing and maintaining good health. Love and trust do wonders to the wellness of our little ones. Many parents today, especially the fathers, have reduced ourselves to a "father Christmas". We deceive ourselves that as long as we are providing, paying the bills etc., then we are done with our role at home. I suggest that it is time we get home, throw away the jacket and sing some songs with our children. They will love it to see Mum and Dad playing together with them. Their joy is health to you as parents. Remember to start and end each day with family prayers by the fireplace. It is said that the family that prays together stays together. Kind, cheerful, encouraging words will prove more effective than most healing medicines. These will bring courage to the heart of the despondent and discouraged. The happiness and sunshine brought into the family by kind acts and words will repay the effort tenfold. Home should be a place where cheerfulness, courtesy and love abide; and where these graces dwell, there will abide health, happiness and peace. No matter how humble, there is no healing environment on Earth like a happy home.

Friend's social health

Many Africans are known for community and extended family social life. It is sad today that this communal social life is dying. No wonder we are having more depressed people today than in the days of our fathers. If you limit your family just to the two of you, maybe with just a child and a dog, soon it will backfire on you. Having genuine friends and relatives whom we can share our sorrows with in time of need, is a remedy and a half. Yes, we need wisdom when sharing our worries and challenges with relatives, church friends or the so-called best friends. Only share your burdens with men and women of wisdom who will encourage and give you sound advice for your particular problem. This will prevent feelings of depression which may result in deterioration of health if you choose to keep issues to yourself. Above all, stay connected with our Benevolent Creator and always put your trust in God. Remember the song in Psalms 103:2,3 "Bless the Lord, O my soul, and forget not all His benefits: who forgives all thine iniquities; who heals all thy diseases."

28. Relationships and Wellness

The quality of our relationships, to a large extent, determines the quality of our health and wellness. I have discovered that it is not just the quantity of our relationships, but also their quality that counts. It is not just how many people we know, how many people we say "hi" to each day. Rather, it is about developing healthy relationships that count. I am talking about relationships that can help us to grow physically, mentally and spiritually. They do matter to our health.

Relationships are most nurturing and therapeutic when we take the time to form that kind of bond. A sense of belonging makes people feel cared for, loved, and valued. It provides social comfort and a sense of control throughout life's unexpected twists and turns. One person in a crisis is a tragedy. Two people in a crisis constitute a support group. The more challenges we face, the more we need other people. Those who lack social ties have an increased risk of dying from coronary heart disease, stroke, cancer, respiratory diseases, gastrointestinal diseases and all other causes of death.

When family and friends pull together for the ones they love, something remarkable occurs. Grace happens. Healing takes place. It may not always be a physical healing; it may be just emotional or spiritual. But it is healing nevertheless. Social health is one of the most powerful predictor of health and longevity. People classified as lonely and isolated have more chances of suffering from chronic diseases as compared to those in happy relationships.

More friends can mean fewer illnesses. Happy relationships are known to boost our immune system. On the other hand, negative social interactions can weaken the important functions of the immune system. The immune system is less effective when one is in conflict with a spouse or companion, even when one is otherwise unhappy. Lack of connection has been found to reduce suppressor T-cells and is associated with recurrence of some illnesses.

Many studies have shown that happily married individuals live longer, with lower mortality for almost every major cause of death, than those who are single, separated, widowed or divorced. God knew the value of relationships from the very beginning. He spent six days filling the earth with plants and creatures of all kinds for Adam to enjoy. But that was not enough. Though Adam had a garden paradise abounding with an incredible variety of living things, he needed something more. And God knew just what that was. "The Lord God said, 'It is not good for the man to be alone. I will make a helper suitable for him.'" (Genesis 2:18). Living creatures surrounded Adam, but he was still alone deep inside. His soul held a vacuum. God used Adam's rib to create the first woman. He could have fashioned her from the dust of the ground, as He did Adam. Or He could have made her from nothing. The basic picture of a healthy relationship that comes to us out of Eden is that of two people clinging together, two people giving themselves to each other. In a world full of self-absorbed people, it is easy to develop our own little self-contained universes: my personal space, my boundaries, my needs, my limits. We are not nearly as dependent on others as we used to be. And that can sometimes be a good thing. But it sometimes leaves us more isolated and self-satisfied. Because we invest less in the relationships that really count, we find ourselves emptier. Our marriages and friendships need some great kind of commitment today. We find healing and nurture only when we invest time and energy in developing good relationships. Meaningful relationships can develop only when we open ourselves up to others. Only to the degree that we become honest and transparent before them will we find nurture and healing.

Let us start today to appreciate our spouses, parents, relatives and friends – one day at a time. Take the challenge to be a good and caring husband, wife, parent or friend. Give and it will come back to you in full measure. Do not sit on the corner waiting to be loved. Take the initiative and enjoy a measure of good health.

PART VI
HEALTHY MIND

29. *Healing the Broken Heart*

"A merry heart works as good medicine but a broken spirit dries up the bones," said the old wise King Solomon. A broken heart is one deadly illnesses that our conventional medicine has little to offer against. Many people are dying silently in their homes with grief and those around them do not even know what to do about it. Grief that causes depression can destroy one's immune system much faster than most feared diseases. One may lose appetite, fail to sleep meaningfully, lose interest in life, and poor health follows as a result. Left unchecked, it can manifest itself as a fatal illness that can cut life even in the form of sudden death.

Feelings of loss and grief can be experienced after we lose someone or something we care about. It can be the death of a loved one, loss of a relationship or a job, a change to your way of life, or loss of important possessions. The grief you experience in these instances is not an illness – it is a normal response to a life event that everyone must face at some point. It takes time to adjust and to learn to live our life without that person, thing or way of life. But in some cases it can be devastating, causing a loss of direction, affecting our relationships and our work.

Mending a broken heart and regaining happiness is not always a miracle, it is a choice and it takes effort and exercise. One step in overcoming grief is having the right perspective of it. We need to remember that feelings of grief are temporary. "Weeping may remain for a night, but joy comes in the morning." (Psalm 30:5). It is never easy to rid oneself of unhappy memories and impressions, but if you wish to regain your health through happiness, then you must do your utmost to forget. Happiness can then take root and a healthy, joyful spirit will provide the best conditions for making and keeping your body healthy. Another important step in overcoming grief is to share your worries with others, especially those who have the ability and wisdom to offer words of encouragement in trying times. Avoid spending time alone and meditating upon the sad things you are going through. Turn your eyes to the wonderful Creator. Trust in divine (God) intervention brings health, healing and hope.

If, however, some sorrow strikes you down, face things bravely with determination to overcome it. Eventually you will reach the place where the warm sun of peace and happiness will once again soothe or even heal your pain completely. Always look ahead with optimism. Life is a series of problems, when one problem is over another one is about to take its place. But remember even among the thorns there are beautiful roses growing. At times these roses may die among the thorns but when the right season comes, they blossom again. There are wonderful things in life that we can always be joyful about, even when our lives are going through the most difficult times.

Should death rob you of your loved ones, try not to be overwhelmed by inconsolable grief. Prophetic words have been written, which promise us a time when there will be no more sorrow, when pain and death will no longer exist. These are not empty illusions. The God of life will put a stop to evil and destruction and the resurrection of the dead will become a reality. This faith in a happier future brings a warm glow of comfort and hope to our hearts. Nothing can strengthen our morale as much as the thought of the restoration of all things to a state of perfection, the way they used to be at the beginning. True, the superficiality of our lives and the cares of day to day living are apt to obscure our understanding of such matters. We think that things have always been and always will be the same. We cannot think of a time when blood will no longer be spilled, when swords will be turned into ploughshares, spears into pruning knives and man will no longer learn the art of war.

Happiness is soothing balm for a sick heart and the best remedy for a wounded spirit. Even when you lose all that you thought was worth living for, or when a once trusted friend deserts you, you will still find that happiness is inexhaustible, once you know where and how to find it. Happiness is to know your savior. The heart of Man will find no rest until it finds its Maker – God.

30. Mind Power and Health

It is easier to accept the news that your liver is not functioning well. But for someone to say your mind is not functioning well, no matter how true that can be, it is an insult. The thing is that there is no difference between you and your mind. You are as healthy as the state of your mind. Positive thinking and positive emotions have a profound effect on promoting and maintaining optimum health. To quote a popular phrase, "the mind is a terrible thing to waste." There are many studies demonstrating the power of the mind. The mind directs the operation of the autonomic nervous system and its neurotransmitters as well as the endocrine system and its hormones for metabolic regulation. Neurotransmitters play an important role in emotions and behaviour. Endorphins are neurotransmitters that are the body's natural relievers. The mind has many well-established and somehow unknown effects on the well-being of your body. The happier you are, the more endorphins you produce.

The mind can rule and modify bodily functions. We reflect what we think. A perfectly balanced mind can handle and detoxify a great burden. When you have a mind and a nervous system that are free of anxiety, worry, fear and are in a state of love, all cells within the system are then in a balance and harmony. Cells in harmony can eliminate and rebuild with great ease. Part of a mental purification programme is to express, let go, feel joy, love without conditions, and forgive. This takes some effort for most of us, as there are many moods involved with changing wrongs that need to be righted and forgiving those who have done wrong things against us.

An open and accepting mind, supplemented with sincere and humble heart, is the fast-track way of receiving this state of unconditional love. Unconditional and thorough love is found in the selfless seeking of truth. This kind of love can free you of the mental stress that compromises your ability to achieve optimum health. It is very important to get your mind and heart in order to experience the highest level of vibrant health.

The power of the mind is considered in some health approaches, but has not been fully embraced by many conventional medical institutions and practitioners. Indeed there is inseparable linkage of the mind to your body and heart in order to experience the highest level of vibrant health at the physical level.

Positive attitude

Looking to the positive, as in seeing the glass half full versus half empty, promotes health for you, your family, and your planet. Your perceptions and views shape the content and character of reality.

Attitude shapes your experiences of health. Viewing yourself at different stages of health versus labelling yourself with diseases and related conditions is a health at the mental level. Today you find many people calling themselves diabetics, hypertensive, etc. The names may sound nice but they are very depressive as they keep on reminding you of the pain you are going through.

Positive emotions

Positive emotions nourish the body while negative emotions are harmful to your body. Love, joy, trust, hope, and forgiveness as opposed to anger, sadness, suspicion, despair, promote health and can reverse disease processes. Seeing yourself in the desired state of health generates the internal energetic and metabolic processes necessary for attaining the physical manifestations of your mental visualisation. This is one of the pathways to wellness.

Support group

An environment that promotes a positive outlook can promote positive health benefits. Developing relationships that support your health philosophies and strategies enhances your realisation of desired health goals. Joining a walking club, a healthy cooking group or a prayer band at your church can be very therapeutic.

Prayer

Communication at the highest level of your being, with the divine power, promotes health beyond limited man-made remedies. This gives wholesome rest to your mind for the accomplishment of needed changes in your lifestyle. Prayer enhances and fortifies your life, taking health beyond physical and mental boundaries. It helps us to reach the highest levels of health and personal development. The mind plays a pivotal role in total health of the body. The mind is nourished by a pure and healthy body and through meditation and positive emotions. For optimum health at the mind level, our prayers and wishes must be harmonised with positive thoughts and actions.

31. The Healing Power of Music

If harsh, clashing sounds such as those made by machines get on our nerves and can damage our health, it is easy to believe that harmonious music would do just the opposite for our wellness. The right sort of music definitely has a beneficial effect on our state of health. There is a lot of noise called music which does more harm to our health than good.

The lullaby a mother or grandmother sings to child is a good example of how a soft melody can have a calming effect. On the other hand; is it not true that the loud blare of pop music coming from a neighbour's open window, when one is trying to relax and rest, has just the opposite negative effect? How many troubled hearts have been smoothed by listening to works of great composers of good, inspiring music? Even the twittering of birds is often able to disperse worry and anxiety to such an extent that those who see no solution to their troubles return home from a walk in the woods, comforted and strengthened, hardly realizing from what source the power came. A crying child may stop wailing just by the singing sound of a bird in the garden hedge. The anger is forgotten and the little face smiles again. It is not surprising that intelligent healers all over the world assert that music has a soothing influence on their patience when under stress and in pain. It relaxes cramped muscles, improves the function of the glands and influences good digestion, which is directly dependent on glandular secretions.

The choice of music

There is a lot of noise in town that goes under the name of music. It goes without saying that not every sort of music has the same effect. Some lovers of soft music might think that it is strange that classical music has the best effect on some sick people, especially if the music contains the message of hope. Music for the sick must be chosen just as carefully as medicine, even with regard to the "dosage", so that its healing powers can work properly. It is not wise for someone who is sick to be listening to music which is very noisy, rough and with a negative message. It is sad sometimes to see people while driving their beautiful cars listening to music that can only remind them of their old terrible days. You hear negative statement like "we are here to suffer", "I am a dead man", etc. Such kind of songs often contain messages about poverty, war, and sometimes death. As your brain starts absorbing these negative messages you start meditating about your lost loved ones who died many years ago. Remember every thought that is generated in your mind affects you emotionally and physically. Good music has power to inspire hope and healing to the broken heart. Bad music can turn a healthy individual into a patient. When people change the kind of music they listen to, their general wellness changes accordingly. The behaviour of a child may change just by changing the kind music the child is exposed to. We should bear in mind the principle that strong stimulants are destructive but weak ones vitalize. Great care should be taken that someone suffering from a grave disease and others with an increased heartbeat are only exposed to soft, harmonious music, which will be of greater benefit to them than fast, exciting sounds. I have also found that soft spiritual music with messages of hope like those contained in most church hymns is therapeutic. Such music has power to lift one's spirit above their challenges. They begin to see a God in their mind who is greater than their challenges and who is able to deliver them from a deadly situation. Such an experience is not just an empty illusion, but it is a connection between man and his maker. Today not everything that goes under the name of gospel music is healing music. Some gospel hits we hear today can do more harm to the sick person if the rhythm is rough, noisy and sometimes without a real message in it. Remember it is the song that inspires, not the drums.

32. Health and Spirituality

A well balanced, healthy diet nourishes your body. A nourished body, in turn, enriches the foundation for the growth of love and peace, which supports the optimum health of your mind. Positive thoughts and emotions then help to nourish the environment for bearing the fruits of unconditional love, which support the health of your spirit. History demonstrates that faithless societies become so corrupt that they cannot survive. Belief is characteristic of science as well as religion. All great civilizations have been founded on religious beliefs and moral values leading to an orderly society. Belief in spiritual values is a strong motivator to treat others well and to develop peaceful relationships. Studies indicate that those in regular spiritual practices who meet with a faith community live longer, live better, and are far less likely to have a stroke or heart attack. Faith can empower you to overcome stress and destructive habits. Trust and reliance in a loving God gives the ability to enjoy a healthful lifestyle. Complete belief in God permits Him to fill our lives with outrageous health!

Spiritual health keeps our entire being in balance. It provides the healthy soil that can prevent us from being overweight and overbearing. Just as fruit and vegetables are the staples for supporting our physical health, unconditional love and forgiveness are primarily staples for supporting spiritual health. Peace, joy, humility and wisdom are the nuts, seeds, grains and legumes that round out a complete whole food diet that supports our spiritual health.

As we develop a relationship with our Creator, we experience a new and improved body, mind, and spirit. As we selflessly share our newfound pearls of health and vitality with our neighbours, we improve the health of ourselves, as well as our neighbours and our planet. Trusting in God who created us enables the harmonious integration of body, mind and spirit. The earthly goal of physical health, which is temporal, is transcended to spiritual health, which is eternal.

Practice makes perfect. It is important to regularly spend some quiet time for the awakening of our inner mind and spiritual self. Daily Bible study, prayer, and service to others are among the most powerful spiritual food known to man. With the daily distractions of today's fast paced life, daily focus on our spiritual side will guard our immune system against the ever-increasing health challenges we face.

Nature teaches many lessons regarding nurturing and healthy living. By observing, studying and applying the powerful laws of nature to our lives, our spiritual enrichment will overcome the boundaries and mysteries of physical limitations. I like to start all of my personalised health plans with the first and most important element, namely, "Spend special time in prayer daily". God can do everything and when we pray to him, we can do everything through His grace. A trusting relationship with the Creator empowers every aspect of our lives and enables us to achieve the fullness of health.

Love is probably the most universal principal underlying most of our different belief systems. Love's mysterious healing energy uplifts us personally and improves our social relationships. It is powerful enough to "heal" the planet.

Our faith, beliefs and hopes affect our health. A loving, all-powerful, all-knowing Creator God is the focus of true health and wellness. Trust in God and reliance on a loving powerful God gives us the ability to enjoy a healthful lifestyles. Complete belief in God permits Him to fill our lives with complete health.

In our world we are surrounded by challenges. Sometimes they are small; sometimes they are big and can seem totally overwhelming. No matter what we face today or tomorrow, experiencing the transformational power of a loving, trusting God can have a profound and positive effect on us. God has expressed His desire to be by our side through every challenge. When we hurt, He hurts with us. He longs for us to trust Him with our challenges, to look up to Him and cling to His strong hand. He longs for us to rest in His loving arms. He will give us strength, courage, peace and complete health.

PART VII
THE PATH TO WELLNESS

33. Seven Tips to Cut Medical Costs

Have you ever seen rich people begging? Yes, from one doctor to another, begging to have their health restored. This precious treasure called "health" rules our happiness. However, do we wait for illness and pain to knock at our door before we think about our health? Today, the whole world has become a huge hospital. It is time for us to do something! Discover the causes of sickness and learn how to prevent them, especially those conditions that are potentially preventable. There are people who blame fate for their poor health, or they blame God or the devil; but sometimes the real cause of illness is the transgression of nature's laws of hygiene, diet and lifestyle. The most common cause of chronic diseases is a lifestyle contrary to the principles of nature. Sedentary lifestyles, incorrect eating habits, drug abuse, use of tobacco, alcohol or other stimulants are some of the underlying factors of modern day chronic diseases.

Our happiness is closely related to our health. We should consider its importance, for God wishes to give us wisdom so we can avoid sickness and He wants to help us regain our lost health: "Beloved I pray above all things that you may prosper in all things and be in health…" 3 John 2.

First Tip

Drinking eight glasses of water a day between meals will help to detoxify the system. We should drink the first two glasses on an empty stomach. A daily shower stimulates both the blood circulation and the nervous system. It cleanses the pores so toxins can be eliminated and contributes greatly to the health of your body.

Second Tip

We should sleep at least 8 hours a day (children require more). Sleep strengthens the nervous system, promotes cell production, aids the secretion of hormones, especially the ones related to growth and helps the body to function correctly. Furthermore, a weekly day of rest is a blessing, both for the body and the soul. In places where people live longer they have a tradition of daily rest and weekly rest like the centenarians of Loma Linda in California, U.S.A.

Third Tip

Be temperate; one should be temperate when eating, at work and in all activities – sexual, intellectual, etc. Temperance means using the good things in moderation and avoiding the bad ones. Even healthy food, if eaten in excess, can be detrimental to our health. We should leave the table feeling that we could eat more. Digestion starts in the mouth, so food should be chewed well. Avoid the temptation to swallow chunks of food. Remember, we do not have teeth in our stomachs.

Fourth Tip

Eat the best food. The body cannot convert junk food into healthy food in our body. We need to choose food not just because it looks and tastes great. Choose the food that will nourish your system, rich in vitamins, minerals, complex carbohydrates, adequate protein and essential fatty acids. An old adage says, "Man should eat to live, not live to eat. The one who eats to live will enjoy good health but the one who lives to eat will burst."

Fifth Tip

Walk! Walk! And walk! Exercise strengthens your body and increases your enjoyment of life. Have daily active outdoor exercises if possible. Aim for at least 30 minutes of exercise a day. Walking is the safest exercise and one of the best. Physical activity combats stress, restores energy, improves sleep and strengthens bones.

Sixth Tip

Expose yourself to fresh air. Air out your home daily and sleep in a room with adequate ventilation. Keep your lungs healthy by taking frequent deep breaths. Walk outdoors when possible, even in winter. Fill your house and surroundings with green plants that absorb carbon dioxide and increase oxygen.

Seventh Tip

Trust in God. A life of quality and fulfilment includes spiritual growth and development. Love, faith, trust, and hope are health-enhancing and they bring rewards that endure. Trust in God brings all healing – physical, mental, emotional, and spiritual.

We cannot be safely guided by the customs of society. The chronic diseases that are becoming a pandemic in our communities today are mainly due to common errors directly related to lifestyle, hygiene and eating habits. Some people are suffering due to ignorance while others are just careless. Either way, one day we will harvest what we sow, either good health or chronic sickness.

34. *Attitude and Healthy Life*

Your attitude influences your health and even impacts the progression of disease. A positive outlook is a gift you give to yourself; it comes as a result of choosing good thoughts also known as positive thinking. God designed each of us to be different, special, unique, and wonderful – but having a negative outlook is not in His plan. A negative outlook switches off the lights of hope. It changes love to hate, and peace to stress. A positive outlook does just the opposite. It turns on the lights, ignites love and allows our heart to focus on possibilities, not problems. God made us to be positive and His example sets the standard. Remember, anything that happens in your mind, the entire body sympathizes with.

Live a life of Hope

I have seen many people recovering faster from deadly chronic diseases because of positive thinking. Positive thinking is based on blessed hope. Hope that, even though your life may be going through rocks, something good is going to happen. It is hope that keeps one's face smiling despite going through pain or trials. It makes sense that, if our thoughts and beliefs can affect us in such powerfully positive ways, they can also affect us in negative ways. This fact provides strong encouragement to choose positive thoughts and beliefs. Positive thinking profoundly affects your total well-being. What we believe about our health, impacts our health. There is a physiological connection between thoughts and health. Our thoughts even affect our destiny. Watch your thoughts, they become your words; watch your words, they become your actions; watch your actions, they become your habits; watch your habits, they become your character; watch your character, it becomes your destiny. Because our thoughts shape who we are, it is vitally important that we are careful with what enters our minds. It is important for us to think about what we are feeding our minds through television, movies, music, radio, and the internet.

Be grateful for your health

Another important part of your outlook is the expression of gratitude for whatever you have. Thanksgiving is a primary ingredient of optimism and a positive outlook. Right now, start making a mental list of what you are grateful for. It can be people or things or whatever. Just start listing them in your head. By doing this, you are counting your blessings. It is as simple as that! Every day, we are either counting or discounting our blessings. Research has shown that people who regularly listed what they were thankful for experienced higher levels of optimism, alertness, enthusiasm, determination, attentiveness and energy than those who did not. Grateful people enjoy higher levels of positive emotions, life satisfaction and vitality than do pessimists. They experience less depression and stress, too. Grateful people do not deny or ignore the negative aspects of life; they just rise above them. Optimistic and grateful people are also more empathetic and are considered more helpful and generous by the people in their social networks. In short, your attitude and outlook can make a big difference in the quality of your mental and physical health. You cannot always change your circumstances, but you can change your attitude towards them, and sometimes that makes all the difference in the world.

Forgive to live

Another essential component of positive outlook is forgiveness. You have to be willing to forgive and to let go of the wrongs done to you. Holding on to hostilities will result in stress, which can weaken the immune system and increase the risk of heart attack. On the other hand, possessing a spirit of forgiveness can actually reduce the same risk. The apostle Paul wrote, "And be kind to one another, tender hearted, forgiving one another, even as God in Christ forgave you." (Ephesians 4:32, NKJV). You see, if we hold on to grudges and hurts, then our hearts sicken, our souls shrivel, and eventually our bodies will physically suffer as well.

35. Starting a Healthy Lifestyle

Many people today would like to change their lifestyles just for the health of it. Nothing is better than that; we need to invest in our health. But remember we are all individuals with unique capacities and requirements. Before making any changes it is important to have a basic understanding of how your body works and what is best for you based on your lifestyle, activity level, known genetic weaknesses, and desired health goals. Many of the stressful effects on your body should be understood and avoided as much as possible. It is important to learn, develop a well thought-out health plan, and then put it into practice. You will need to develop your own personalised health strategy.

You own your health and, as such, you have enormous latitude in choosing the strategy for optimising your personalised, dietary regimen. Certainly, this does not mean that everyone has to become a nutritionist or health professional. It is important, however, to develop a basic understanding of body functions and nutritional requirements. Once armed with this understanding, you may even opt to work with a qualified health practitioner or practitioners who are sympathetic to meeting your requirements.

The more skills and strategies you have available, the greater your opportunity for reaching your desired health goals through proper nutrition and lifestyle. If you hire a carpenter to build a house, you are much more likely to have expectations and requirements met if the carpenter has a full complement of tools as opposed to just a hammer and a pair of pliers. Our bodies perform best with grains, fruits, vegetables, nuts and seeds, etc. All other foods are tolerated based on our individual requirements and capacities. Common sense tells us that we should honour these principles in accordance with our desired physical, mental, emotional, and spiritual goals.

Care must be taken when making a transition from a compromised lifestyle to a more healthy one. When your body undergoes major changes in a short period of time, it can often experience discomfort. We often crave for things to which we have become addicted. Your body, however, becomes addicted to good habits just as it does to poor practices. It will take time to re-programme your habits and lifestyle so be patient and do not give up.

The discomfort a person generally feels during a lifestyle transition is sometimes referred to as a "healing crisis". Your body always strives to improve, repair, and continually cleanse itself. Given a new healthful environment, your body tends to release stored waste and repair your metabolic system at a faster rate than the elimination organs can handle. Feelings of nausea, headaches, light-headedness, and flu-like aches and pains are not uncommon. It is important to understand this phenomenon and work through it to a healthful conclusion. Working with these discomforts while you employ the appropriate nutritional and support strategies will yield significant benefits. These symptoms are part of the balancing process that is necessary for optimum health.

For major changes in diet, strong motivation and willpower may be required. In many instances a more gradual change in "bite-sized" pieces is a better approach. Even doing this, you will make significant progress in a reasonable period of time. It is important to remember that a changed diet and lifestyle do not occur overnight. It will take some time to reclaim your optimum health. It could take from a few months to several years for major improvements to occur. Don't try to change everything in one afternoon, but make a quick progressive change and make it fun. The investment in your personal health development and maintenance will repay you attractive dividends. Prayer is a very powerful enabler in any dietary and lifestyle programme. God can do anything, and when we pray to Him, He will assist in our efforts because He desires for us to be in good health and it is one of His greatest blessings.

36. A Balanced Lifestyle

As a Nutritional Therapist, one of the challenges I face from day to day is to educate people how to live a balanced lifestyle. In our communities we have two common groups of people. They are those who are careless with their lifestyle and those who have gone to the other extreme of becoming health fanatics. Sometimes when we are running away from danger, there is also a danger of going to the extreme. From the health point of view, both fanatics and the careless ones are in danger. What we need is a balanced lifestyle.

Living a balanced lifestyle means choosing the good things in moderation, and avoiding what is harmful. Healthy choices are a key to a balanced life. Think of how a radio equalizer works. As we use the equalizer to balance the highs and lows of music, so we can use the power of our choices to avoid extremes.

Making good choices requires a balanced approach in all that we do. Even a good thing can be overdone. If a person exercises so much that they do not have time to spend with their family and friends, the exercise has become out of balance and can cause problems in other areas. Yes, it is possible to have too much of a good thing. And if we choose to include good things in our lives but fail to eliminate the negative things, we are also doing ourselves a disservice. For example, the benefits to our cardio-respiratory system when we eat oatmeal for breakfast may be minimized or eliminated if we also eat a lot of high cholesterol foods like sausages and fried chips at the same time.

It is a good idea to use honey instead of sugar as a sweetener, but that does not mean too much honey is safe for our bodies. Moderation is key to a balanced lifestyle. I always encourage people to eat more fruits and vegetables. However, it is important to discourage the tradition of consuming too much fruit of the same type in one go. It is common, especially in developing countries, to see someone eating a whole bunch of 20 bananas or a basin full of mangos, especially when they are in season. The best way of eating fruits is to have two or three different fruits at a meal time. For example you may choose to have one apple, one banana and one orange at breakfast time. Consuming too much fruits or sugarcane at once can raise our blood sugar, making us feel dizzy and weak a few minutes later due to the action of the hormone insulin. High fibre diets are excellent, but remember you do not have to eat that brown rice to the point where you struggle to breathe. Eat smaller portions at meal times.

37. Fighting the Winter Blues

Winter time gives us a break at least from those hot months. It is time we start making use of our blankets, our favourite warm suits and jerseys. There is less work for gardeners due to winter rain showers. What a wonderful time to grow those plants that normally do well only in winter. For firewood and charcoal sellers it is time for better cash flow than any other time of the year. But not everything is wonderful in winter. During the winter season you may also experience sniffles, stuffy nose, aches of the cold, as well as the outright misery of influenza. I call these winter blues. Did you know that good nutrition and lifestyle can help to prevent the flu plague?

Good nutrition

Eat more fruits and vegetables. Many of us do not like eating fruits in winter which is the opposite of what we must be doing. Especially fruits that are rich in vitamin C like lemons, oranges, apples, pineapples, kiwi, grapefruit, etc. These fruits are immune boosters and excellent in fighting infection. Herbal teas like Rooibos, Echinacea and Hibiscus are flu fighters as opposed to caffeine drinks which may lower your resistance to the winter blues. The body's defence system will be excited if you include vegetables like broccoli, spinach, cauliflower, sprouts, butternut, among others. Every time you eat the greens you are giving yourself a pack of minerals and vitamins needed by the body to fight infection. Nuts and seeds are another group of food not to be ignored. They are rich in zinc, which is one of the soul foods for your immune system. Pumpkin seeds, ground nuts, Sunflower seeds are the most common ones in most developing countries. Other nuts and seeds like almonds, flaxseeds, and cashews are just as good. Use less fatty foods and cooking oils. Where possible cut down refined foods like jam, sweets, ice creams, chocolates, white bread, cakes and foods that are rich in sugar.

Go for a walk

During cold seasons it is easy to hibernate by spending our time indoors and many hours by the fireplace or electric heater. But it is important to get out for a walk outdoors. Oxygen-rich fresh air from outside is therapeutic and can easily fight off infection. If your house is surrounded by trees, you are more blessed. Walking for about 30 minutes to 1 hour everyday can make a big difference. Brisk walking encourages deep breathing and optimal oxygen intake, much better if it is done as first thing in the morning.

A healthful lifestyle

A good lifestyle can greatly assist in maintaining a strong immune response. The body is the physical temple and it is to be honoured. It is wise to look after it with excellent care and never abuse it for any reason. This means: obtain plenty of rest and sleep, at least nine hours daily. Learn the habit of going to bed early. The hours before midnight are worth at least four times the benefit of sleeping after midnight, be in bed by 9pm if possible. Stress is another immune destroyer, look at the sunny side of life, count your blessings and always rejoice in your wonderful creator. Laugh a lot. It is said that laughter is good medicine. "A merry heart is good medicine, but a broken spirit drains your strength." Proverbs 17:22.

38. *Health, Healing & Hope*

Many people today are searching for good health, some for healing and others for hope. Health is a treasure. Of all temporary blessings that we have in this life nothing can surpass good health. Many people don't appreciate the good health they have until the day they lose it. I have seen people laughing at those who are trying to live a healthy lifestyle, calling them health fanatics. But as time progresses they become victims of lifestyle diseases and begin searching for healing. Human beings are very strange. They spend their health trying to make money and later they spend all their money trying to gain health. I am sure you have seen people spending all their pension money on hospital bills. The cost of managing lifestyle diseases is very heavy and it pays to prevent than managing the curse. You may have known people who ended up selling, cars, plots, land trying to raise money for treatment of chronic diseases.

Health

It's easy, change your lifestyle and enjoy the measure of good health. Bless yourself with natural foods. Whole grains, nuts, fruits and vegetables prepared in a simple way, provides both nourishment and healing to our bodies. Add to the good diet some physical activity, not as an event but a lifestyle. You will find walking for 30 minutes every morning makes a big difference. People who do exercise everyday have a stronger immune system than their sedentary peers. As a bonus, if you are physically fit, your muscles do burn more fats when you are resting. Your mental health will be at its optimum if you have a good dosage of physical activity. Never neglect the importance of water. Ever wonder that most people will never forget to check water in their car's engine, but they can hardly remember the last hour they took a glass of water for themselves. The law of harvest is just as true as the law of gravity. If something goes up we know that at one point it will come down. And what you sow is what you reap. Some of these chronic conditions like diabetes, blood pressure, cancer, arthritis, gout, etc. are not necessarily the illness that we catch, but rather what we harvest after many years of unhealthy lifestyle. If the laws of health are not observed sickness will follow. Ignorance is not an excuse either. Whether you know how to prevent these curses or not you will still reap what you sow.

Healing

If you happen to be one of the people suffering from lifestyle diseases don't lose hope either. You can suppress the promotion and even the progression through lifestyle modification. I have seen a number of patients at my Wellness Clinic kissing diabetes goodbye, reversing the first and second stage of cancer, reclaiming back a life without blood pressure problems through our lifestyle medicine program. Imagine living a life of praise to your benevolent creator without the need to remember taking chronic medication. True healing is holistic. It involves personal health awareness of physical, mental and spiritual health. You need to be educated on how to live a lifestyle that will restore your health. It doesn't matter how you have lived in the past. You can make a new start today and have a brand new end. To achieve this goal you may need therapeutic coaching, guidance and inspiration. Remember you are not alone; you are simply joining the crowd of people who have decided to take responsibility of their health.

Hope

It's good to have good health and it's wonderful to experience healing but we all need hope. I remember counselling a lady who was also a prayer warrior. She did not blame God for her poor health condition. Instead she accepted responsibility that her poor lifestyle through ignorance was the culprit of her misfortune. Yet she believed that her redeemer lives and because God lives she will live too. She decided to cooperate with her creator by adopting a healthy lifestyle. Never have I seen a person recovering from a lifestyle condition faster like the way I saw it happening with this lady. Yes, hope may not always end in healing. One musician wrote a song some years ago he said "we have this hope that burns in our hearts, hope in the coming of the Lord". For sure the day is coming when the final act of healing will take place. God will take His children home, where there will be no more illness, no sorrows neither death. The hand of man will finally touch the hand of God.

ABOUT THE AUTHOR

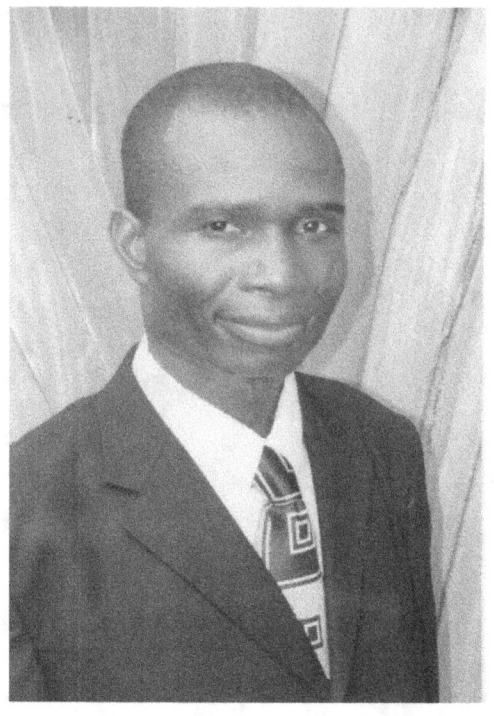

Gandy Madzalo is a Naturopathic Nutritional Therapist, Wellness Educator, trained in Hydrotherapy, Phytotherapy, Therapeutic Massage and Wellness Coaching. He teaches and coordinates health and wellness educational programs to both corporate and communities.